Praises for Thi
The Bragg Heal

D0595293

These are just a few of the thousands of testimonials we receive yearly, praising The Bragg Health Books for the rejuvenation benefits they reap – physically, mentally and spiritually. We look forward to hearing from you also.

Thanks to Bragg Health Books, they were our introduction to healthy living. We are very grateful to you and your father.
– Marilyn Diamond, co-author, *Fit For Life*
– Best Seller for 40 weeks

The Bragg Healthy Lifestyle with Fasting has changed my life! I lost weight and my energy levels went through the roof. I look forward to my fasting days. I think better and am a better husband and father. Thank you Patricia, this has been a great blessing in my life. Also, we enjoyed your important health sharing at our "AOL" Conference.
– Byron H. Elton, former VP Entertainment, Time Warner AOL

Thank you Patricia for our first meeting in London in 1968. You gave me your *The Miracle of Fasting* Book, it got me exercising, brisk walking and eating more wisely. You were a blessing God-sent. – Reverend Billy Graham

---

When I was a young gymnastics coach at Stanford University, Paul Bragg's words and example inspired me to live a healthy lifestyle. I was 23 then; now I'm over 63, and my own health and fitness serves as a living testimonial to Bragg's wisdom, carried on by Patricia, his dedicated health crusading daughter. Thank You Both!
– Dan Millman, author, *Way of the Peaceful Warrior*
• *www.peacefulwarrior.com*

Bragg Super Power Breathing and Lifestyle makes the weak strong and helps make athletes Olympic winning champions.
– Bob Anderson, famous stretching coach • *Stretching.com*

Just by paying attention to breathing and health, you can access new levels of health and relaxation that will benefit every area of your life.
– Deepak Chopra, M.D. • www.deepakchopra.com

Praises for This Book and The Bragg Healthy Lifestyle

Paul Bragg saved my life at 15 when I attended the Bragg Health Crusade in Oakland. I thank Bragg Healthy Lifestyle for my long, healthy, active life spreading health and fitness.
– Jack LaLanne, Thankful Bragg follower to 96 1/2 years

Thanks to Paul Bragg and the Bragg Books, my years of asthma were cured in only one month with The Bragg Healthy Lifestyle Living and *The Miracle of Fasting*.
– Paul Wenner, Creator of the original Gardenburger

The Bragg Healthy Lifestyle and brisk walking (3x daily) for 20 minutes after meals, helped eliminate my diabetes! My whole body, circulation, feet and eyes have all improved. Thank you, may God continue to bless your Crusade.
– John Risk, Santee, CA

As a youth I had a learning disability and was told I would never read, write or communicate normally. At 14 I dropped out of school and at 17 ended up in Hawaii surfing. My road to recovery led me to Paul Bragg who changed my life by giving me one simple affirmation: "I am a genius and I apply my wisdom." Bragg inspired me to go back to school and get my education and from there miracles happened. I have authored 72 training programs and 40 books and love to crusade around the world thanks to Paul Bragg.
– Dr. John Demartini, Dynamic Crusader
Star in "The Secret" • *www.DrDemartini.com*

I had the opportunity to sit next to Patricia on a flight from Dallas to Los Angeles. Her honesty about my weight and health really inspired me to make a life change. One year later, I am 85 lbs. lighter and heart rate cut almost in half. Patricia you helped save my life! – Mike Ableman, TX

Our great-grandmother will turn 100 in two weeks. She still kayaks, gardens, and shovels her own snow covered driveway. For over 80 years, she had one recipe for life: 2 Tbsps apple cider vinegar and 1 tsp. of honey mixed into water. This is the secret, she says, to a life worth living!
– The Alvina Sharp Family, Chanhassen, Minnesota

Praises for This Book and The Bragg Healthy Lifestyle

Your dad, Dr. Paul Bragg, IS the FATHER of the Natural Health Industry and the entire Natural Health Movement. Everything that has been done in natural health and physical culture since has been based on the pioneering vision and principles articulated by Dr. Paul C. Bragg. He gave us all our direction!
– Dr. William Wong, Texas

I love Bragg Books and *The Miracle of Fasting*. They are so popular and loved in Russia and Ukraine. I give thanks for my health and super energy. I just won the famous Honolulu Marathon with the all-time women's record!
– Lyubov Morgunova, Champion Runner, Moscow, Russia

I have known the Bragg Books for over 30 years. They are a blessing to me and my family and to all who read them to help make this a healthier world. – Pastor Mike Macintosh, Horizon Christian Fellowship, San Diego, CA

I've been reading Bragg Books since high school.
I'm thankful for the healthy lifestyle and admire their health crusading to make this a healthier world!
– Steve Jobs, Creator – Apple Computer/iPods

Thanks to Bragg Fasting Book & Healthy Lifestyle, we are healthy, fit and singing better and staying younger than ever!
– The Beach Boys • *www.TheBeachBoys.com*

In 1975 I was diagnosed with coronary heart disease. I followed the Free Bragg Exercise Classes and Lectures at Fort DeRussy lawn, Waikiki Beach, six days a week. Thirty-one years have passed, I am now 84-years young thanks to *The Bragg Healthy Lifestyle*. – Helen Risk, R.N., Hawaii

---

Bragg Books were my conversion to the healthy way.
– James F. Balch, M.D., *Prescription for Nutritional Healing*

Improper breathing is a common cause of ill health. Changing your breathing patterns can affect and improve you mentally, emotionally and physically. – Andrew Weil, M.D. • www.DrWeil.com

Praises for This Book and The Bragg Healthy Lifestyle

How I beat cancer, obesity, diabetes, strep and three herniated disks and excruciating pain? The answer was changing to the Bragg's Healthy Lifestyle! It changed and saved my life! I had full recovery and also lost 70 lbs. I received a new life and that is just the beginning because my manhood returned that was lost to diabetes – now that's exciting! On my trip to Honolulu, Hawaii I visited the famous free Bragg Exercise Class at Waikiki Beach. I became so regenerated with a wonderful new viewpoint towards living my healthy lifestyle that I now live in Hawaii. I'm invigorated with new energy for life and living! My new purpose for living is to help others reclaim their health rights! I also want the world to join The Bragg Health Crusade. I am deeply thankful to Paul and Patricia for my happy, healthy life! – Len Schneider, Hawaii

---

Thank you Paul and Patricia Bragg for my simple, easy to follow Bragg Healthy Lifestyle. You make my days healthy! – Clint Eastwood, Academy Award Winning Film Producer, Director, Actor and Bragg follower for over 60 years

---

Patricia Bragg is a dedicated Health Crusader and she shared her Bragg Healthy Lifestyle with millions of our radio listeners. Thank you Patricia. – Host George Noory, *Coast to Coast Radio*

We get letters daily at our Santa Barbara headquarters. We would love to receive a testimonial letter from you on any blessings, healings and changes you experienced after following The Bragg Healthy Lifestyle and this book. It's all within your grasp to be in top health. By following this book, you can reap more Super Health and a happy, longer vital life! It's never too late to begin. Studies show amazing results that were obtained by exercise with people even in their 80's and 90's – pages 117 to 118. You can receive miracles with healthy nutrition, fasting and exercise! Start now!

Daily our prayers & love go out to you, your heart, mind & soul with love.

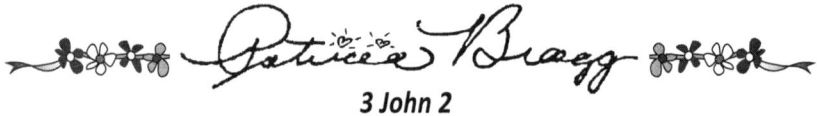

3 John 2

Miracles can happen every day through guidance and prayer! – Patricia Bragg

Patricia Bragg Books

Building Powerful NERVE FORCE & Positive Energy

Reduce Stress, Worry & Anger

PAUL C. BRAGG, N.D., Ph.D.
LIFE EXTENSION SPECIALIST
and
PATRICIA BRAGG
HEALTH CRUSADER & LIFESTYLE EDUCATOR

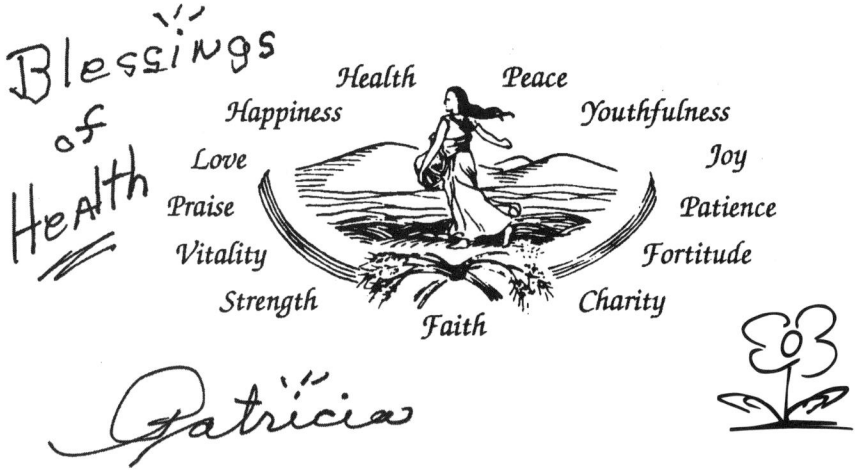

BECOME

A Health Crusader – for a 100% Healthy World for All!

---

www.PatriciaBraggBooks.com

Building Powerful NERVE FORCE & Positive Energy

Reduce Stress, Worry & Anger

PAUL C. BRAGG, N.D., Ph.D.
LIFE EXTENSION SPECIALIST
and
PATRICIA BRAGG
HEALTH CRUSADER & LIFESTYLE EDUCATOR

Copyright © by Health Science ~ All rights reserved under the International Copyright Union. No portion of this book may be reproduced or used in any manner without the written permission of the publisher, except by a reviewer who wishes to use brief quotations for magazine, newspaper, web, blog, radio or television program.

Visit our website:
www.PatriciaBraggBooks.com

Sixteenth Edition MMXXI
ISBN: 978-0-87790-091-7

Library of Congress Cataloging-in-Publication Data on file with publisher

Published in the United States
HEALTH SCIENCE
7127 Hollister Avenue, Suite 25A, Box 249, Santa Barbara, CA 93117
Toll-Free: (833) 408-1122

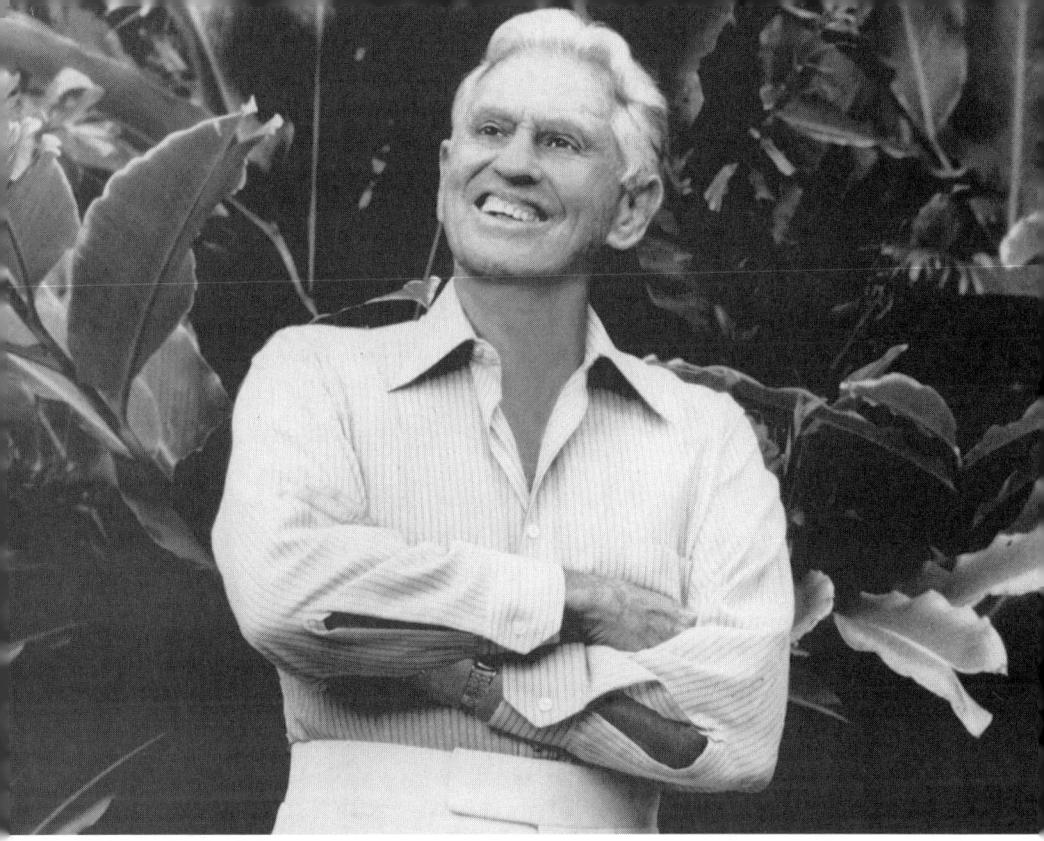

PAUL C. BRAGG, N.D., Ph.D.
World's Leading Healthy Lifestyle Authority

Paul C. Bragg's daughter Patricia and their wonderful, healthy members of the Bragg *Longer Life, Health and Happiness Club* exercised daily on the beautiful Fort DeRussy lawn, at famous Waikiki Beach in Honolulu, Hawaii. On Saturday there were often health lectures on how to live a long, healthy life! The group averaged 50 to 75 per day, depending on the season. From December to March it can go up to 125. Its dedicated leaders carried on the class for over 43 years. Thousands visited the club from around the world and carried the Bragg Health and Fitness Crusade to friends and relatives back home.

Your body is a non-stop living system, in constant motion 24 hours daily, cleaning, repairing, healing and growing. – Patricia Bragg

To maintain good health, normal weight and increase the good life of radiant health, joy and happiness, the body must be exercised properly (stretching, walking, jogging, biking, swimming, deep breathing, good posture) and nourished with healthy foods. – Paul C. Bragg, N.D., Ph.D.

Cautionary Note and Disclaimer

The information provided here is for educational purposes only. Any decision on your part to read, listen and use this information is your personal choice. The information in this book is not meant to be used to diagnose, prescribe or treat any illness. Please discuss any changes you wish to make to your medical treatment with a qualified, licensed health care provider.

If you are taking medication to control your blood sugar or blood pressure, you may need to reduce the dosage if you significantly restrict your carbohydrate intake. This is best done under the care and supervision of an experienced and qualified licensed health care provider. Anyone who has any other serious illness such as cardiovascular disease, cancer, kidney or liver disease needs to exercise caution if making dietary changes. You should consult your physician for guidance. If you are pregnant or lactating, you should not overly restrict protein or fat intake. Also, young children and teens have much more demanding nutrient needs and should NOT have their protein or fat intake overly restricted.

The information presented in this book is in no way intended as medical advice or a substitute for medical counseling. It is intended only to provide the opinions and ideas of the authors. It is sold with the understanding that the authors are not engaged in rendering medical, health or any other kind of professional services in this book. The reader should consult his or her medical doctor, or any other competent professional, before adopting any of the suggestions in this book, or drawing inferences from it.

The authors disclaim any responsibility for any liability, loss or risk, personal or otherwise, which is incurred as a consequence, directly or indirectly, of the use and application of the contents of this book.

Please consult your physician before beginning this program, and use all of the information the authors suggest in conjunction with the guidance and care of your physician. Your physician should be aware of all medical conditions that you may have, as well as medications and supplements you are taking.

Building Powerful NERVE FORCE & Positive Energy

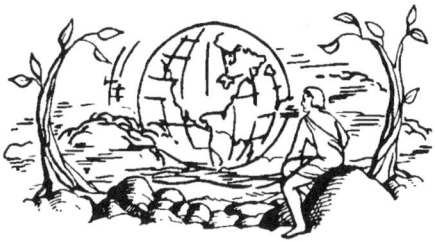

To preserve health is a moral and religious duty, for health is the basis for all social virtues. We can no longer be as useful when not well.
– Dr. Samuel Johnson, Father of Dictionaries

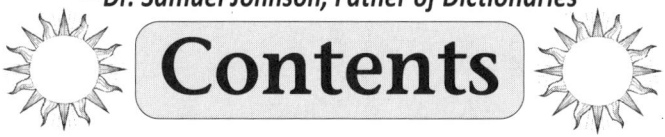

Contents

Praises for The Bragg Healthy Lifestyle . . . . . A-D

Chapter 1: What is Nerve Force? 1

What is Meant by 'Nerves'? 1
Your Body's Command Center (list) 1
The Three Forms of Nerve Force (list) 2
Equilibrium of the Nervous System (graphic) 3

Chapter 2: Building Powerful Nerve Force 5

Nerve Force is Your Vital Key to Life 5
Paul C. Bragg Pioneered New Way to Health 6
The Secret of Nerve Force 6
Nerve Force is the Key to Vital Living 7
"Bad Nerves" Are Dangerous 8
There is No Mental Health Without Powerful Nerve Force 8
Depleting Our Reservoir of Nerve Force 9
The Danger Signals of Low Nerve Force (list) 9
A Healthy Lifestyle is Best Remedy for Nervous Disorders 11
Live as Mother Nature Intended You to Live! 11
Happiness and Love Are Simplicity 12
Love and Survival 12
The Art of Long, Healthy, Happy Living 13
Build Your Own Nerve Force 14
This Is Your Life To Love and Protect 14

Open my eyes to see clearly the wonders of thy teachings. – Psalms 119:18

Contents

Chapter 2: Building Powerful Nerve Force (continued)

Worry and Stress Are Killers 15
Suicide Rate Soaring Among All Ages 15
A Healthy Lifestyle Prevents Suicide 16
From Nervous Breakdown To Health Buildup 16
Keep Your Nerves Healthy and Strong 18
Two Sides of the Shield – Physical and Mental 18
A Strong Mind in a Strong Body 19
Make Your Body Worry-Proof 20
There is No Reward For Worry 21
Help with Panic Attacks 21
Good Posture Promotes Healthier Nerves 22
Where Do You Stand? Posture Chart (graphic) 23
Start Building Your Nerve Force Today! (list) 24
Your Stress Scale Test 26

Chapter 3: The Importance of NERVE FORCE 27

Nerve Depletion: A Lack of Nerve Energy 27
Nerve Depression: Decreased Energy Flow 28
Nerve Tension: Excessive Nervous Energy 29
Recognizing and Avoiding Hypertension 29
High Blood Pressure in Adolescence 31
Lower Your Blood Pressure Naturally 31
Biofeedback Empowers You to Relax 33
Self-Pity is a Nerve and Energy Robber 34
Self-Talk and Even Write to Yourself 34
Positive Health Statements To Use (list) 35
Some Need Professional Help 36
Nerve Force is Powerful and So Important 36

Contents

Physical and Mental Deterioration 37
Impaired Metabolism Causes Body Imbalance 37
Post-Traumatic Stress Disorder – "PTSD" 38
Nervous Disorders Upset the Stomach 38
Millions Suffer From Nervous Indigestion 38
Heartburn = Higher Risk For Cancer 39
Depression and Stress May Affect Diabetics 39
Nerve Depletion Promotes Constipation 40
For Easier-Flowing Bowel Movements (graphic) 41
Feed Your Nerves – Don't Destroy Them! 41
Avoid Junk Foods and Harmful Stimulants 41
Your Gut Influences Your Emotional Health 42
Living The Bragg Healthy Lifestyle May Reverse Cellular Ageing! . 43
Millions Suffer From Nerve Exhaustion 44

Chapter 4: Spiritual Health Promotes Physical Health. 47

First Step to Powerful Nerve Force: Meditation & Prayer 47
Simple Techniques of Meditation & Prayer 48
Meditation and Prayer Helps Master Life 49
You Are What You Think and More 49
Your Life Is The Miracle of Miracles 50
To Over-Rest is To Rust 50
Build *"The Will to Win"* in Your Life 51
You Need Inspiration To Guide Your Destiny 52
Faith and Vision Create Miracles 52
Therapeutic Use of Forgiveness 53
Let Mother Nature and God Inspire You! 54

When you sell a man a book you don't just sell him paper, ink and glue, you sell him a whole new life! There's heaven and earth in a real book. The real purpose of books is to trap the mind into its own thinking. – Christopher Morley

Contents

Chapter 4: Spiritual Health (continued)

There Are Six Basic Fears (list) 55
Fear of Sickness 56
Fear of Poverty 56
Fear of Old Age 57
Fear of Criticism 58
Fear of the Loss of Love 59
Fear of Death 60
The River of Thoughts – Positive or Negative 61
Faith Versus Fear 61
Overcoming Fears 62
Inspiring Words Bring Miracles 62

Chapter 5: Sound, Peaceful, Recharging Sleep 63

Second Step Towards Powerful Nerve Force 63
Relaxed – Deep Sleep Must be Earned 63
Your Mattress Is Your Best Sleeping Friend (graphic) 64
Dreams Can Reflect Past and Present Life 65
Books Can Be Your Teachers & Relaxers 66
Outwitting Insomnia 67
Natural Ways to Cure Insomnia (list) 67
Fitness Trainers Say Days Off Benefit Fitness 68
Food and Drink – Their Effects on Sleep (list) 68
Simple Ways to Keep Stress Levels Low (list) 69
67% American Adults Are Sleep Deprived 69
Are You Getting Enough Sleep Lately? 69

I know the sunny side of life. My Nerve Force gives me the power to radiate sunshine in the gloomiest of times. – Paul C. Bragg, N.D., Ph.D.

Laughter is inner jogging, good for your body and soul. – Norman Cousins

A laugh is just like sunshine. It freshens all the day. – Heart Warmers

Contents

Try Lemon Balm Tea for a Night So Calm. 70
Good Sleep is the Cornerstone of Health 70
Healthful Tips for Sound Recharging Sleep (list) 71
Lifestyle Suggestions that Enhance Sleep (list). 73
Relief for Snorer in the House 73
Stanford's Suggestions for Improving Sleep (list). 74
The Luxury of the Siesta. 75
Try Power Nap For Miracle Recharge. 75
How to Have Deep, Sound, Relaxed Sleep 76

Chapter 6: Natural Healthy Food 77

Third Step Towards Powerful Nerve Force 77
The Bragg Healthy Lifestyle Eating Habits 77
Healthy Plant-Based Daily Food Guide (graphic & list) 78
Bad Nutrition – #1 Cause of Sickness (photo) 81
You Are Exactly What You Eat and Drink. 81
Millions Suffer Vitamin B-Complex Deficiency 82
Folic Acid Helps Protect the Blood 83
High Homocysteine Can Cause Alzheimer's, Diabetes
and Heart Health Problems 83
B Vitamins & Folic Acid Are Heart Protectors 84
Foods Rich in the B Vitamin Family (list) 85
Your Nerves Need Plenty of Calcium. 85
Calcium Deficiencies Cause Nervous Habits 86
Calcium Content Chart of Some Common Foods 87
Benefit From Natural Foods Rich in Calcium 88
Milk is Not a Good Source of Calcium. 88
Calcium Can Help Tame PMS 88
Locations in the Body Where Osteoporosis Hit the Hardest . . 89
Some Body Signs of Potassium Deficiency (list). 90

Contents

Chapter 6: Natural Healthy Food (continued)

Nature's Miracle Phytochemicals Help Prevent Cancer (chart) . . .91
Food and Product Summary. 92
Enjoy Super Health with Natural Foods (list). 92
Enjoy Lighter, Smaller Vegetarian Dinners 93
Avoid These Processed, Refined, Harmful Foods (list) 94
Beware: Why "Modern" Wheat is Bad for You 95
Keep Blood Sugar Levels Low and Healthy (list) 96
Increase Your Stamina and Go Power 97
Stamina-Boosting Foods and Nutrients 97
The Stamina Balance. 97
Boost Your Memory 98
The Brain – Memory Boosting Diet 98
Nutrients and Herbs to the Rescue. 98
Plant-Based Protein Chart 99
Vegetable & Fruit Juices Contain Mother Nature's Water 100
The 75% Watery Human (graphic) 101
Water is the Key to All Body Functions 102
Allergies and Dr. Coca's Pulse Test 103
Most Common Food Allergies (list) 103
My Daily Health Journal (copy page) 104
Dr. Charles Attwood – Great Health Crusader. 105
Dr. Attwood's Tips for Low-Fat Shopping (list) 105
Dr. Kellogg's Famous Menus 106-107
Bragg Health Beverages & Nutritious, Delicious Recipes . . 108-109
Benefits from The Joys of Fasting (list). 110

True wisdom consists in not departing from nature, but molding our conduct according to her wise laws. – Seneca

Our habits, good or bad, are something we can control. – Dr. E. J. Stieglitz

Contents

Chapter 7: Exercise Your Body 111

Fourth Step Towards Building Nerve Force 111
Walking Helps Remove Emotional Tensions 112
Expert Advice on How to Exercise (list) 113
What Miracles Exercise Can Do For You 113
Benefits that Daily Exercise Can Bring You (list). 114
Exercise Promotes Health & Youthfulness 114
Enjoy Exercising – It's Healthy and Fun! (photo). 115
Enjoy Exercise and Jogs for Longer, Healthy Life (photo) . . . 116
Iron Pumping Oldsters Triple Muscle Strength (photo) 117
Amazing Health & Fitness Results in 8 Weeks. 118
More Muscles Linked to Longer Life. 119
The Benefits of Being Fit and Healthy 119
Exercise is the Best Fitness Conditioner 120
The Miracle Life of Ageless Jack LaLanne (photo). 120
Macfadden – Founder of Physical Culture (photo) 121
Healthy Heart Habits for Long Vital Life (list) 122

Chapter 8: Correct Breathing 123

Fifth Step Towards Powerful Nerve Force 123
When You Breathe Deeply You Live Longer and Healthier . . . 123
The Lower Respiratory System (graphic) 124
Path of Breath & Mechanics of Breathing (graphic) 124
Shallow Breathers Self-Poison Themselves. 125
What is Diaphragmatic Breathing?. 126

Breathing deeply, fully and completely energizes the body, calms the nerves, fills you with peace and helps keep you youthful. – Paul C. Bragg

---

The heart that loves is always young. – Greek proverb

To relax quickly SMILE, then take a good deep breath and then slowly exhale.

Contents

Chapter 8: Correct Breathing (continued)

How to Practice Diaphragmatic Breathing 126
Advantages of Diaphragmatic Breathing (list) 126
Control Nerves with Diaphragmatic Breathing. 127
Long, Slow Diaphragmatic Breathing Leads to Long Life! . . 128
Deadly Smoking – Health Hazard to Avoid. 129
Deadly Smoking Facts – Reasons to Stop! (list) 130
Quit Smoking – See the Difference it Makes! 131
Heimlich Maneuver Jumpstarts the Lungs 132
Heimlich Helps Save Drowning Victims. 132

Chapter 9: Bathing & Circulation 133

Sixth Step Towards Powerful Nerve Force 133
Cold Water on the Skin is Important. 134
Special Shower Builds Healthy Circulation 134
Cold Water Swimmers Are Fit and Ageless (photo) 135
Warm and Hot Baths also Have Their Place 136
Five Hidden Dangers in Your Shower (list) 137
Use Shower Filter to Remove Toxins. 137
Showers, Toxic Chemicals & Chlorine. 138
You Get More Toxic Exposure from a Shower (graphic) 139
Swimming is a Great Nerve Force Builder 140
Enjoy Energy from Gentle Sunbathing. 141
Gentle Sunbathing Works Miracles! 142
Enjoy Sunshine for Super Health 142

Throughout my life with my strong Nerve Force, I have received strength, enthusiasm and purpose of mind, body and soul.
– Paul C. Bragg, N.D., Ph.D., from "Awaken Health and Happiness," 1937

A good laugh is sunshine in a house. – William Makepeace Thackeray

We shall never know all the good that a simple smile can do. – Mother Teresa

Contents

Chapter 10: Keep Your Emotions Under Control . . . 143

The Seventh Step to Building A Powerful Nerve Force 143
Follow These Stress Reducing Guidelines (list) 143
Avoid Arguing, Teasing, Bullying & Nagging 145
Shun Constant Suspicion 146
Reap the Rewards of Smiling 146
Happy Feelings Are Internal Smiles 147
Instant Mood Lifters (list) 147
Remove Negative Chips Off Your Shoulders 148
Paul C. Bragg Practiced Thought Substitution 149
Send Your Worry to the Winds 150
Make Your Own Sunshine & Happiness 151
Have an Attitude of Gratitude! 151

Chapter 11: Healthy Relaxation 153

The Eighth Step to Building A Powerful Nerve Force 153
Relaxation is a Healthy, Soothing Feeling 154
Feelings, Tension & Relaxation Create Heartbeat of Life . . . 155
There Are No Magic Cures 157
Ten Great No-Calorie Stress Busters (list) 158
The Benefits of Full Yoga Breathing (list) 158

Chapter 12: Enjoy Life! 159

The Ninth Step to Building A Powerful Nerve Force 159
Learn to Live Joyously with Yourself 159
Slow Down and Enjoy Each Day! 159
Healthy Body = More Peaceful Mind 160

Doubt destroys. Faith builds. – Robert Collier

What really matters is what you do with what you have! – Shirley Lord

It's never too late to be what you might have been. – George Elliot

Contents

Chapter 13: The Biochemistry of Mental Health. . .161

Nervous Problems Are Epidemic! 161
Nutritional Therapy for Hyperactive Children 162
Here is Dr. Feingold's Basic Health Program (list) 162
About Chronic Fatigue Syndrome – CFS 163
Dr. Balch's Health Suggestions to Combat CFS (list) 164
Avoiding Metabolic Syndrome. 165
Diet is Vital to Developing Intelligence and Brain Cells 166
"Junk S.A.D. Foods" Starve the Brain and Body 167
Vitamins & Minerals to Treat Mental Issues. 168
Magnesium – Essential for Healthy Nerves 169
75% of Adults Deficient in Magnesium 170
How Much Magnesium Do You Need? 171
Calcium: The Other Half of the Dynamic Duo 171
Chelation Therapy Cleanses Arteries. 172
There's Many Ways to Stop Anxiety & Depression (list) 172
Take an Active Role in Your Own Health Care 173

Chapter 14: Relief for Nervous Tension & Anxiety . . 175

Here's One of the Main Causes of Nervous Tension 175
Chronic Depression May Lead to Cancer. 176
Link Between Stress and Cancer. 176
Importance of Normalizing Blood Pressure 177
Hypertension Can Be Prevented. 178
Combating Depression, Stress & Anxiety (list) 178
More Stress Relieving Suggestions 179
Soothing Remedies for Tension Headaches (recipes) 180
Foods Can Trigger Stress-Related Migraines. 180

The natural healing force within us is the greatest force in getting well.
– Hippocrates, Father of Medicine, 400 B.C.

Contents

Headache Acupressure Points (graphic) 180
Scientists Reveal Certain Foods Can Alter Moods 181
SAMe: A Safe Natural Antidepressant 181
St. John's Wort Relieves Depression 182
Depression & Transcranial Magnetic Stimulation. 183
Enhance Mood and Mind with Vitamin B1 183
Help For Bipolar Disorder Mood Swings 183
More Natural Remedies for Mood Swings 184
Ginkgo Helps Depression, Stroke & Brain Recovery 185
Candida Linked to Chronic Fatigue, Bloating & Nausea . . . 185
The Fast Growing Healing Revolution 186

Chapter 15: Alternative Health Therapies 187

Acupuncture, Chiropractic, Colon, Skin Brushing. 187
Homeopathy, Naturopathy, Osteopathy, Reflexology, Water . . . 188
Alexander, Feldenkrais, Reiki, Rolfing, Tragering,
Massage & Aromatherapy 189
Massage: Self, Shiatsu, Swedish, Sports 190
Control & Extend Your Health & Lifespan! 191
From the Authors 192
More Praises and Testimonials. 193-196

Bragg Photo Gallery. 197-206

INDEX 207-214

Bragg Health Books / Patricia & Paul Bios . . 215-219

START BEING HAPPIER, SMILE AND LAUGH MORE – it's up to you! Healthy actions speak louder than words and can elevate your mood if you feel depressed. Take a brisk walk in a natural setting and practice slow, deep breathing – it helps you sort out and solve problems. Spend time with children, it simplifies life and puts everything in perspective. Find comics in the newspaper or something funny to read and laugh. If someone is upset, try to analyze the situation from that person's perspective. As often as possible make yourself smile and laugh; it opens blood vessels in the back of your head to physically lift your mood. Choose to be happy in spite of circumstances. No one "makes" you happy – it's an inner attitude that sparkles from within.

Why My Father & I Wrote This Book

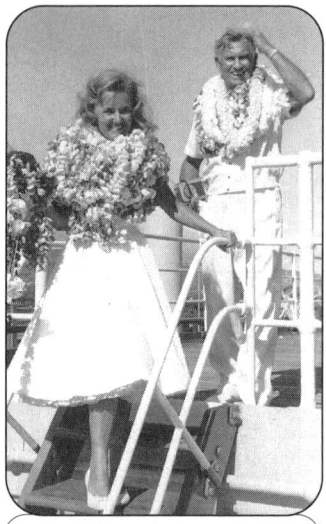

World Health Crusaders
Paul C. Bragg and daughter, Patricia

Let us share with you our experiences with Powerful Nerve Force versus Nervous Fatigue. My father knows what it is to be so exhausted that every cell of your body seems to cry out with extreme weakness! He was once so ill and weak that he couldn't raise his head from a pillow. That changed because he changed his lifestyle.

Dad learned how to rebuild his Powerful Nerve Force the Natural Way and lived to be a great-great-grandfather with a vast storehouse of energy. We enjoyed our ageless, tireless bodies and enjoyed our busy life and got more accomplished than ever – yet we still had time to indulge in our many athletic hobbies. We've hiked tall mountains and could play a fast game of tennis with people young enough to be our great-grandchildren! We swam and lifted weights 3 times a week. We rode our bikes or jogged for miles at a time, then wrote books and at times traveled off on the Bragg Health Crusades around the world to spread health.

This book outlines our Bragg Building Powerful Nerve Force Program. It can change your entire life! You will learn how to master your life with new zest for living and how to change nervous exhaustion into inexhaustible energy! You can build a new life for yourself if you follow our program faithfully . . . because your life and energy flows through your nerves! We can help, but it's your life and it's up to you!

Bragg Healthy Lifestyle Plan

- *Read, plan, plot, and follow through for supreme health and longevity.*
- *Underline, highlight or dog-ear pages as you read important passages.*
- *Organizing your lifestyle helps you identify what's important in your life.*
- *Be faithful to your health goals daily for a healthy, long, fulfilled life.*
- *Where space allows we have included "words of wisdom" from great minds to motivate and inspire you. Please share your favorite sayings with us.*
- *Write us about your successes following The Bragg Healthy Lifestyle.*

What is Nerve Force?

What is Meant by 'Nerves'?

The popular expression "nerves" can actually mean Nerve Exhaustion or lack of Nerve Force. To ask, "What is Nerve Force?" one might as well ask, "What is Electricity?" Both are just as intangible. **We know that Nerve Force is the Vital Force of Life, a mysterious energy that flows from the nervous system to give life and energy to every vital organ. Sever the nerve which leads to any organ and the organ will cease functioning.**

The wonderful structure we term the Nervous System consists of millions of cells which act as reservoirs of Nerve Force. The amount of stored energy represents our Nerve Capital. Every organ works incessantly to keep the supply of Nerve Force in these cells at a high level. Life itself depends more upon Nerve Force than upon the food we eat or even the air we breathe. Without the activating Nerve Force we could neither breathe nor eat!

Your Body's Command Center

It is the health and vitality of the millions of nerve cells that make up your vast nervous system. You need a powerful Nerve Force – stored in the numerous and varied nerve cells composing the nervous system – to attain and maintain the ideal balance for perfect super health. The nervous system consists of two sections controlled by a centralized command center – your miracle brain:

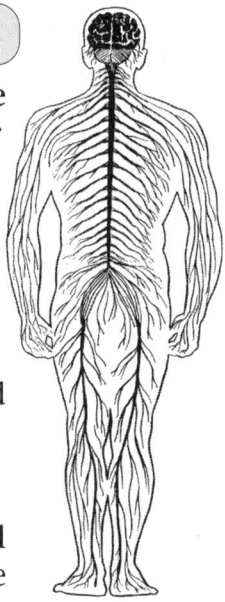

NERVOUS SYSTEM

1. The External Nervous System:

Controls the skin surface and external muscles of the body. It transmits to the brain's command center that governs movements of the arms, legs, head and other external muscles, as well as the skin's sensitivity to heat, cold and injury.

2. The Internal Nervous System:

Known as the Autonomic System – **it has two subsystems, the sympathetic and the parasympathetic. These govern the internal functions of the body (i.e., the vital organs).**

3. The Brain: Acts as clearing house for the entire organism – **the "control room" in which the mind "programs" the whole body's "computer system."** It is interesting to note that according to scientists the human brain has a storage capacity of about 1,000 years.

The Three Forms of Nerve Force

There are three forms of Nerve Force by which the human "network," your nervous system operates:

1. Muscular Nerve Force: This is the Nerve Force that produces our muscular action. A high degree of this force is found in those insects and smaller animals which have tremendous muscular power in proportion to their size. An elephant could jump over mountains and push down the highest skyscraper if it possessed the same degree of Muscular Nerve Force as a flea, ant or small bug!

2. Organic Nerve Force: The activity of our vital organs depends upon this form of Nerve Force. A high level of this Nerve Force produces robust health and the ability to resist disease. This leads to a long, peaceful, healthy life.

3. Mental Nerve Force: Essentially a mental quality, a powerful Mental Nerve Force that produces a keen intellect, good memory, mental endurance and a generally high psychic power. High Mental Nerve Force denotes a well-balanced, healthy person that has good control of their emotions. Stresses, strains and tensions do not plague them since they are the master of their own destiny. Their Mental Nerve Force is so high that they are impervious to petty nagging and other minor irritations which people of lower Mental Nerve Force try to impose upon them.

It's suppose to be a professional secret, but I'll tell you anyway. We doctors do nothing. We only help and encourage the doctor within.
– Albert Schweitzer

No one can drag you down from your high pedestal of bliss-consciousness when your Mental Nerve Force is high! You are never out of mental equilibrium. You are a natural human being who enjoys a constant mental state of bliss. You have mental poise. You live by knowledge and wisdom. You know true contentment and peace of mind and body. Relish it and treasure it!!!

Equilibrium of the Nervous System

In 1588, famous English poet William Byrd expressed it so beautifully in his *Psalms and Sonnets:*

My mind to me a kingdom is;
Such perfect joy therein I find,
That it exceeds all other bliss
that God or Nature hath assigned.

Mother Nature strives for perfect balance or equilibrium. When humans interfere with the balance of Nature they are in for trouble.

There are three main factors which disturb the equilibrium of the Nervous System: *Nerve Depletion, Nerve Depression* and *Nerve Tension*. We will use non-technical terms while discussing these afflictions because we want even the untrained student to understand each aspect of the topic. For example, when we refer to the Nervous System, we're generally alluding to the Internal (inner) and External (outer) workings.

Nerves are Pathways that Carry Vital Info Between Your Muscles, Organs and Brain.

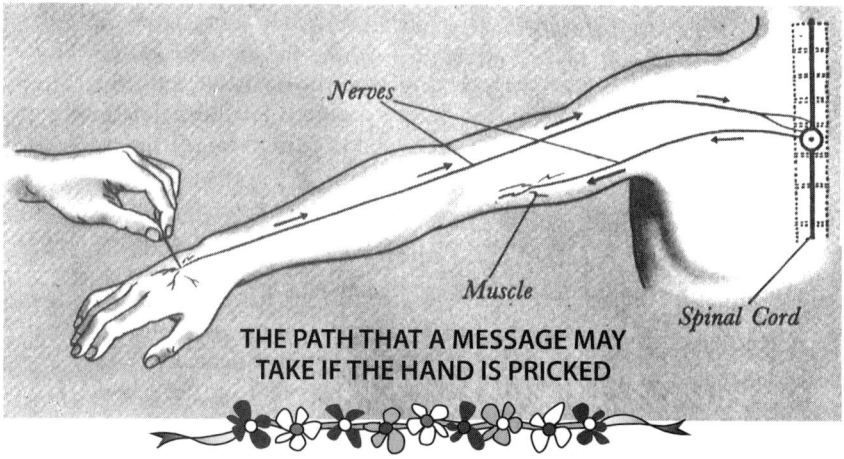

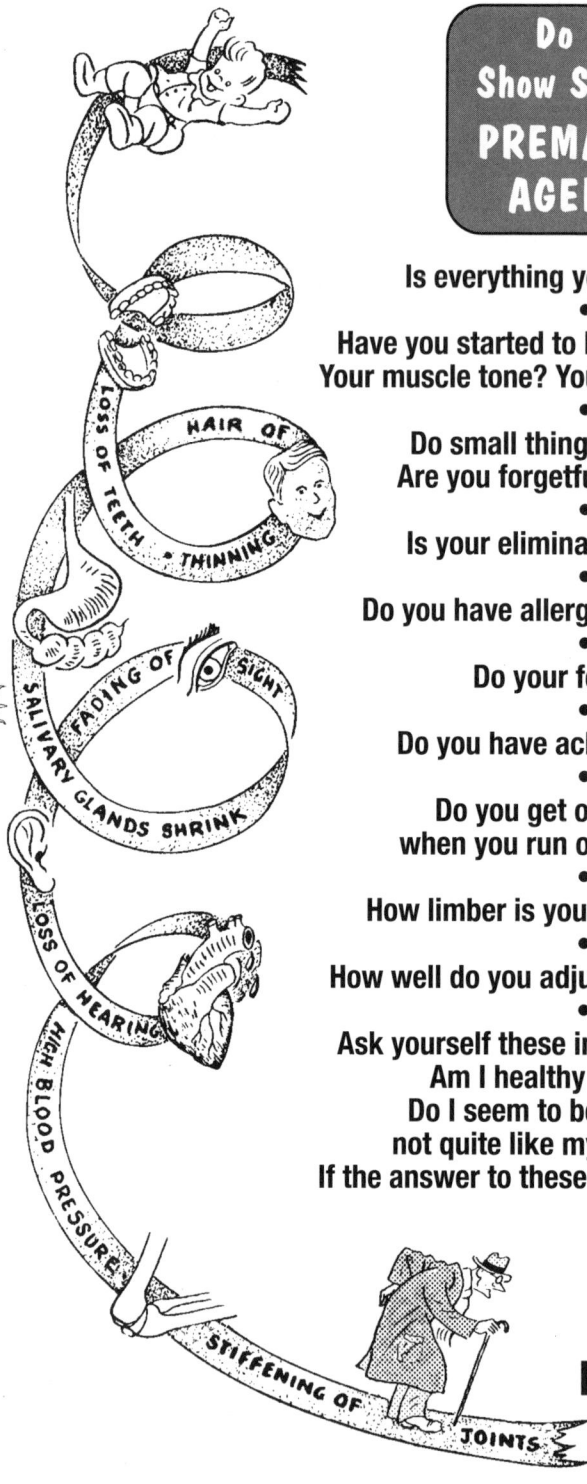

Do You Show Signs of PREMATURE AGEING?

Is everything you do a big effort?

•

Have you started to lose your skin tone? Your muscle tone? Your energy? Your hair?

•

Do small things irritate you? Are you forgetful? Confused?

•

Is your elimination sluggish?

•

Do you have allergies? Joint pains?

•

Do your feet hurt?

•

Do you have aches and pains?

•

Do you get out of breath when you run or climb stairs?

•

How limber is your back and body?

•

How well do you adjust to cold and heat?

•

Ask yourself these important questions: Am I healthy and happy? Do I seem to be slipping and not quite like myself anymore? If the answer to these questions are "Yes,"

START TODAY Living The Bragg Healthy Lifestyle!

Building Powerful NERVE FORCE & Positive Energy

Nerve Force Is Your Vital Key to Life

My father and I loved being Health Crusaders and made no attempt to produce literary classics when writing the Bragg Healthy Lifestyle books. We wrote in simple, easy-to-understand language and presented health facts and wisdom that can be deeply imprinted upon the reader's mind to inspire them to live a healthy life. Our health message is of such vital importance that it should be brought to the attention of every man, woman and youth around the world.

We are living in the age of nerve stress. The terrific strain of the present-day "mile-a-minute rat race" is slowly but surely undermining the very foundations of our existence. Unless we take determined steps now to counter-act this threat, in a few decades we may find ourselves in a world populated with nervous wrecks! We are especially concerned for the American people. Throughout the world sufferers from nervous disorders abound, but sadly it's the American men, women and children who strain their nerves the most.

Our deep interest is in sharing this message of how to have healthy nerves, since each of us is governed by our Nerve Force. I am also interested in this subject because my father was born with highly sensitive nerves. I too have always had high energy, along with sensitive, active nerves. As a young man it became imperative for my father to learn to control his Nerve Force so he could reach his lifetime goal – being a Health Crusader!

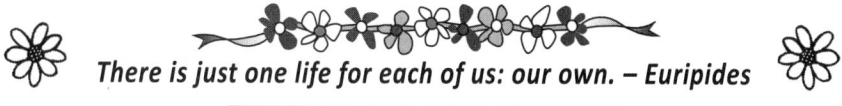

There is just one life for each of us: our own. – Euripides

I strive to be pure and good in all things – in body, mind and soul.
– Paul C. Bragg, N.D., Ph.D.

Good health and good sense are two of life's greatest blessings.
– Publilius Syrus, 42 B.C.

Paul C. Bragg Pioneered New Way to Health

After he had defeated tuberculosis at 18, Dad became intensely interested in healthy lifestyles and fitness and resolved to achieve the highest physical perfection allowed by Mother Nature. The developmental process of his study and practice of Health Culture began with physical exercise and athletics because he believed – as many do today – that muscular strength means health. As the fallacy of this dangerous theory became clear to him, he began to concentrate on scientific nutrition, deep breathing and systematic body-building to repair and renew his physique. He remained always on the alert to find the weakest cog in his body's machinery.

He found the most vulnerable factor in health to be the nerves, the body's governing force. That is where the body is weakest and most sensitive to abuse. We must begin to build up our Vital Nerve Force in the nerves! This statement is not based upon mere theory. **Dad personally supervised Physical and Nutritional Programs for thousands yearly, also teaching thousands of students who attended our Bragg Health Crusades worldwide. The truths of my father's early teachings are now becoming accepted and honored by the top Universities and Health Professionals worldwide.**

The Secret of Nerve Force

Nerve Force is the source of all life! Life itself flows through your nerves – never forget that! When fully supplied with Nerve Force, we are enthusiastic, happy, fit and ambitious. We overcome difficulties and are ready to accept the challenges that life offers. Problems of all kinds become manageable when we are confident that we have Vital Nerve Force to cope with them.

People with powerful Nerve Force cannot be beaten. They rise up again for a new start, no matter how often they might fail. In the end, they win! Thus, 95% of humanity is dominated by the other 5%. It's Nerve Force that does the leading and makes the difference!

When health is absent, wisdom cannot reveal itself, strength cannot be exerted, wealth is useless and reason is powerless. – Herophiles, 300 B.C.

Nerve Force Is the Key to Vital Living

Your health, strength, vitality and endurance are directly measured by the degree of your Nerve Force. It gives you the reserve power that makes life successful and fascinating. The world is full of people with the brains and ability to rise to the top, but who lack the necessary Nerve Force to push them forward. A person's beauty, charm and vivacity are directly related to the Nerve Force that makes them sparkle with radiant health.

Your body is a complicated machine; Nerve Force and physical health are interdependent. Nerve Force is the driving power – but its generation, in turn, depends upon the harmonious activities of the vital organs. Your body is nourished throughout its every part by a vast circulatory system that carries oxygenated blood from your heart and lungs. If an organ is not functioning properly, your blood will not contain the elements necessary to create the right sort of Nerve Force. Your stomach must digest efficiently. The digestion assimilating process must be dependable. The eliminating organs – the bowels, lungs, kidneys and skin – must have tremendous Nerve Force to work efficiently. **The spleen, liver and all the vital organs of the complex blood-making laboratory must all work harmoniously.**

If you arise every morning feeling dull and fatigued, if you are without ambition or goals, if you feel old, worn and dragged-out, or if the future looks hopeless and you feel defeated and helpless, then there's something wrong with your nervous system! Your Nerve Force is depleted and must be renewed! Good News: You don't have to feel this way! Read on – learn how to improve your life!

There is one thing you can do – start rebuilding your vital Nerve Force today! The body is a miraculous self-cleansing and self-healing organism when you give it and Mother Nature a chance. Unfortunately, most people, especially Americans today, are depleting their Nerve Force and are whipping their nerves in a desperate effort to compensate. This only makes everything worse.

Over a 70 year lifespan, your busy stomach processes about 40 tons of food.

Perfect health is above gold; a healthy body before riches. – Solomon, 900 B.C.

"Bad Nerves" Are Dangerous and Are Destroying American Youth and Adults

"Bad Nerves . . ." We hear about them constantly and everywhere! The physician tells a patient, "It's your nerves." Sensitive and highly-strung people complain about their "nerves." Day after day you hear of housewives, blue-collar workers, business and professional people having a "nervous breakdown." You even hear parents say of their child, "He's so nervous, he won't listen to me and I can't discipline him!"

America is a nation of nervous people, a fact known the world over and openly admitted by our own nerve specialists. Our national intensity is directly related to our "mile-a-minute" lifestyle that causes nerve burnout! It's making us the most progressive nation on earth . . . but it's also destroying our health! Our crowded mental institutions prove this. Half of the hospital beds of the country are occupied by people with nervous disorders!

There Is No Mental Health Without Powerful Healthy Nerve Force

The best authorities on mental health say that if mental illness continues to increase at the present rate, in less than a hundred years there will be no one to take care of the mentally ill because everybody will be the victim of some mental disorder! Sounds frightening, doesn't it? Medical records prove it. There are not enough psychiatrists and psychologists to handle the mentally ill today. America is in a sad and deplorable situation!

Millions of people have subnormal Nerve Force and as a consequence suffer from endless organic and physical troubles which make their lives miserable. When people don't have the Nerve Force or basic vitality to meet the pressure which life puts upon them, what happens? Let's take a look. The first thing most people do is to take one of the milder stimulants – such as tobacco, coffee, tea, or cola drinks – to combat their stress. The deeper their Nerve Force reserves drop, the more often they seek out the stronger stimulants – alcohol and harder drugs. It is not long before far too many of them become addicted to some dangerous and powerful drug.

There are many people who consider themselves normal, yet they cannot go through an ordinary day without the use of some kind of pill. At night their nerves are so exhausted that they can't get rest without a sleeping pill! Just watch your TV and note how many pain, sleeping and tranquilizers pills are advertised!

Depleting Our Reservoir of Nerve Force

There are numerous ways we unduly tax our nerves: poor nutrition, lack of oxygen or regular sleep, stress, overwork, anger, worry, jealousy, hate, envy, greed, self-pity, guilt and grief. If we subject our muscular system to excessive strain and consume more Nerve Force than the body can produce, the natural result is Nerve Bankruptcy: complete Nerve Exhaustion and maybe even a nervous breakdown! There is but one malady more terrible than Nervous Exhaustion – its kin, insanity! Those who have endured this know the terrible suffering involved. **Nervous Exhaustion can put a cloud of misery over your life.**

The Danger Signals of Low Nerve Force

When the Nerve Force is low, you can go through life burdened with fear and never recognize its presence. Only a courageous self-analysis will disclose the presence of this universal enemy. When you begin such an analysis, search deeply into your character and be brutally honest with yourself! As you will note, the symptoms of fear and low Nerve Force themselves will work against such honesty.

Even in Australia, total cost of workers compensation claims for stress-related conditions is over $200 million every year!
– BetterHealth.vic.gov.au

Americans fill more than 4.5 billion prescriptions a year.
– Center for Disease Control and Prevention • www.cdc.gov

Yesterday is the past. Tomorrow's the future. But today is a gift . . .
That is why it is called the present.

Who is strong? He that can conquer his bad habits. – Benjamin Franklin

You must collect and redirect your remaining Nerve Force to head-off these danger signals! It's your first step onto the Road of High Health. ***Please Check For:***

1. Indifference: Do you tend to easily accept, without protest, whatever life offers you? Do you lack initiative, imagination, enthusiasm and self-control? Low Nerve Force drains away your ambition, while it's making you mentally and physically lazy, willing to tolerate poverty or a lower standard of living. It also makes you unable to get out of a demeaning situation in your life.

2. Indecision: Are you inclined to let others do your thinking for you? Would you rather be led than make decisions for yourself? A person with low Nerve Force is easily brainwashed because others can control their mind. They can actually become a human robot who does not question anything, even their own actions!

3. Doubt: Do you secretly doubt your ability to do things and as a consequence, also doubt the sincerity of those who want to help you? Low Nerve Force is often characterized by excuses designed to cover up, explain away or apologize for personal failures. It is sometimes expressed in the form of criticism or envy of those who have sparkling health or those who have found success in life.

4. Worry: Are you a chronic worrier? This is a major danger signal of low Nerve Force and can easily lead to a nervous breakdown! Worriers are miserable people, living in a haze of fears. Worrying saps the life out of a person and ages them prematurely. It is an absolute and scientific fact studies show that you can worry yourself into the hospital and an early grave!

If your Nerve Force is low to the point of chronic worry, you will probably say, "If you had my problems, you would worry, too!" That is not necessarily true. Everyone encounters problems as life goes on – often bigger ones than you have encountered. But a person who has powerful Nerve Force does not worry about a problem. They face it objectively and in a calm, logical, practical way they find a solution! Often, after carefully examining a problem and if they are unable to find a solution, they will turn it over to a Higher Power and pray for the answer. **We have seen miracles with prayer and meditation!**

Worrying about a problem will not solve it! It only destroys your health and ages you prematurely. Worry is a killer! **Build a strong Nerve Force and solutions come.**

5. Being Overly Cautious: Do you wait for "the right time" to begin putting ideas and plans into action – until waiting becomes a permanent habit? When Nerve Force is low, pessimism is high. One habitually looks for the negative side of every situation – thinking and talking of possible failure instead of concentrating upon the means of success. This leads to knowing all the roads to disaster, but never searching for ways and means to avoid failure. **Constant procrastination and uncertainty often leads to tension, poor circulation, indigestion, constipation, nervousness, bad breath and a terrible disposition.**

A Healthy Lifestyle is The Wisest and The Best Remedy for Nervous Disorders

Let it be definitely understood that we can't offer any cures for nervous conditions. We do not prescribe, diagnose or treat disease in any way. That is strictly for the doctors. We are teachers instructing people in a Program of Natural Living that will keep their entire body in good physical condition. This program – The Bragg Healthy Lifestyle – includes correct daily habits of eating, exercising, sleeping, breathing, fasting, relaxing, bathing, posture, and even a technique of meditation and prayer for developing control over the mind and body. Everyone who wishes to be free from chronic fatigue and build powerful Nerve Force must have full control of both their mind and body.

Live as Mother Nature Intended You to Live!

One of the dominant themes of this book is a gradual return to a more natural way of living. In your thinking, eating and all of your daily habits, you must strive for simplicity of life. Try to reach a nearness to Mother Nature and make yourself at home with her. When you feel that the same pure forces which express themselves in a beautiful pine tree are manifesting themselves in you, then you have made a big stride toward the ideal life.

Begin to live as Mother Nature and God want you to live. Seek and feel their love and know you can be part of their healthy world-wide family. In your daily meditations and prayers repeat over and over again, **"I am becoming Mother Nature's perfect child." You become one with Mother Nature when you live the natural Bragg Healthy Lifestyle. As you become a part of Mother Nature in body, mind, and spirit, you will soon be able to attain the highest possible Nerve Force!**

Happiness and Love Are Simplicity

Happiness and Love are what we all seek, and when found, life can be heaven on earth! Let's be like children – pleased with simple things! The more we complicate our lives, the more we drain our Nerve Force. With wholesome health and serenity of mind, let us live our lives in tranquility and contentment! Let us find the pure joy of living! Let us love Mother Nature as she reveals herself to us in all her simplicity and beauty! If we live a useful, humble, sane life according to her righteous laws – cultivating happiness and sharing it with those near and dear to us – we will do more than well! The best religion of all is found in kindness, understanding, giving and sharing. The real measure of our sunshine is in the brightness we can kindle in the eyes of others.

Love and Survival

Famous Dr. Dean Ornish (*Ornish.com*), states how you feel emotionally can affect your health physically . . .

In my work with cardiac patients over the last 30 years, I am convinced that love and intimacy are at the root of health and illness; there is such a thing as the healing power of love!

UC Berkeley Scientists studied patients who were undergoing coronary angiography. Those who felt the most loved and supported by family and friends, had substantially less blockage in the heart arteries. These findings are similar in Swedish Research. More than 1,700 men and women between the ages of 29 and 74, were studied for 6 years. Those who were more isolated with low emotional support were four times more at risk of dying prematurely.

Clearly, Scientific Studies have proven that the capacity to nurture and be nurtured – to have a loving heart is a vital link to a long and healthy life!

If we will only let her, Mother Nature will comfort us and bring us joy. Let us try to understand her with our mind and heart and enjoy her with the open and glad hearts of children! To have overall powerful Nerve Force we must learn the great Laws of Mother Nature and live by them. That is what this book is all about. Its purpose is to show you how to live by the Laws of Mother Nature and reap the rewards of Health and Happiness for a long, beautiful life! The kingdom of heaven is within you! Make your heaven here and now!

By trusting in Mother Nature and obeying her laws, understanding your physical machinery and the way to care for it, you can build a powerful Nerve Force that can bring you unbelievable happiness! No matter how low you feel mentally, physically, spiritually and emotionally, know that the body is a self-cleansing, self-repairing, and self-healing instrument. Give your body a chance and its recuperating vital forces can make you an amazing new healthy, happy, fulfilled person!

The Art of Long, Healthy, Happy Living

One of the best recipes for a long, healthy and happy life is just to keep on living by Mother Nature's Laws. Consider each day as a little life in itself and make it as perfect and well-rounded as you possibly can.

What you sow in one period of your life, you reap in another. Live well today so you will have a better tomorrow! Try to be better physically and mentally on your next birthday than you are now. By living supremely for the moment you are investing in a superb life for your future. However, please be aware of yourself! The moment you relax your guard, the enemy is ready to rush in and smite your weak spot. A few may live long and happily without trying to live well and healthfully, but you will live longer, be healthier and happier if you make a conscious effort! **Living for health, longevity and happiness is an art. If you deliberately strive to prolong your life in health and happiness, you may just do so!**

Build Your Own Nerve Force

The reason we told you we offer no magic cures for people with nerve problems is because to build powerful Nerve Force you, and you alone, must do it! It is day to day living and thinking that is important. We will outline our entire Bragg Healthy Lifestyle for you in this book, but we cannot live it for you – nor can anyone else! No one can eat, exercise, fast, breathe or meditate for you. The more you put into this Nerve Force Program, the more good benefits you will reap from it!

Our Program is designed to not only give you powerful Nerve Force, it will also make you a more balanced person physically and mentally. The program is designed to lead you to "bliss consciousness," which simply means getting more out of your life – more peace, serenity and happiness. This is the true joy of living!

This Is Your Life To Love and Protect

You were put here to enjoy life! And though we firmly believe that the kingdom of heaven is within every person, we also believe that you must work to reach that heavenly state of joyful living! We must earn it! It is not handed out on a silver platter. **Remember that what you give to life is what you get from life. The results you will get out of The Bragg Healthy Lifestyle will be in exact proportion to the effort you put into it.**

Nerve Force is the most precious gift of Mother Nature. It means everything – your happiness, your health and your success in life. You must learn all there is to know about your nerves: how to protect, relax, calm and soothe your nerves. In this way, you can rebuild your precious Nerve Force, as you strive to keep yourself healthy, physically and mentally fit.

Life is a gift – open it. A joy – share it. A game – play it. An experience – live it. A dream – make it come true!

"Why not look for the best – the best in others, best in ourselves, best in all life situations? He who looks for the best knows the worst is there, but refuses to be discouraged by it. Life will soon become more pleasant for you and everyone around you." – Rev Paul S. Osumi, Hawaii

The *Archives of General Psychiatry* cites recent studies that show how stress markedly delays wound healing. One study assessed the relationship between the psychological stress and the secretion of pro-inflammatory cytokines – development of local immune responses that are central in the early stages of wound repair. Researchers induced skin blisters on the forearms of 36 women. Those with higher perceived stress scores had lower level of cytokines production, causing slow healing.

Worry and Stress Are Killers

Nerve and stress related diseases occur world-wide. In many parts of the world, decreased physical activity and unhealthy diets are leading to obesity, increased blood pressure, cholesterol and diabetes which leads ultimately to cardiac problems.

Most humans are so full of worry that they believe they can never overcome their miseries. Each day the little bit of Nerve Force they have is dissipated by worrying about their difficulties. The surest way to become a nervous wreck and arrive at a complete nervous breakdown is to worry. Worrying about a problem does not solve it – it only makes things worse. As we said before, you can literally "worry yourself to death." A Hollywood neighbor of ours almost did!

Suicide Rate Soaring Among All Ages!

This woman had multiple serious problems. She suffered with migraine headaches that almost drove her crazy. She was chronically constipated, tortured by insomnia and gas pains. Her husband was an alcoholic. Their two children were wild, uncontrollable teenagers who brought her and her husband nothing but grief. She was worried to the breaking point and had thoughts of committing suicide. Records show in America, thousands resort to suicide to escape from their worries (*cdc.gov*). Sadly suicide rates are soaring among teenagers.

Alcohol abuse and Alcoholism are tragically the third leading cause of preventable deaths in the United States.

No man can violate Nature's Laws and escape her penalties! – Julian Johnson

A Healthy Lifestyle Prevents Suicide

Finally, this neighbor came to our home one evening and told us what she had in mind. Naturally we told her this was a terrible thing to do to herself. We knew she could overcome her problems if she would follow Mother Nature's Laws. We told her that no matter what her worries were, we believed that if she would build her Nerve Force she could find the answers to most of her problems. We also told her that she had attempted to break every law of health and natural hygiene. By breaking these laws she had only succeeded in destroying her own physical, emotional and mental health!

We finally told her that we had no magic cures to offer her. All we could do was give her our complete Nerve Force Program and Bragg Healthy Lifestyle, which both obey Mother Nature's Eternal Laws!

The first thing about The Bragg Healthy Lifestyle we outlined for our neighbor was a fast of 3 days, allowing nothing but distilled water. We told her to leave home and go to some quiet spot in the country where she could enjoy absolute rest during this cleansing, recharge time.

From Nervous Breakdown To Health Buildup

She went to Lake Arrowhead, CA and rented a cozy cabin among the big pines, and went on a complete 3-day distilled water fast. As she flushed the poisons out of her body, she became calmer and was able to see her problems more objectively. **This period of body purification made tremendous changes physically, spiritually, emotionally and mentally in her well-being. Her thinking was fresher, clearer and happier. She could take a overall bird's-eye view of her problems and start solving them, thoughtfully one at a time.**

The alcohol habit is the most harmful to the body and must be stopped! The Center for Disease Control and Prevention states excessive alcohol consumption is the 3rd largest cause of death after smoking and obesity.

Learning is finding out what you already knew. Doing is demonstrating that you know it! Teaching is reminding others that they know it just as well as you! You are all learners, doers and teachers! – Richard Bach

We outlined for our neighbor The Bragg Healthy Lifestyle eating program that eliminates all coffee, soda and unhealthy, devitalized foods. We put her on a healthy vegetarian diet for a full month. We told her to meditate and pray for 30 minutes in the morning and again at night. During these calm meditations she was to repeat the following affirmations, many times at first:

- ***I have mind-heart-soul power to solve all my problems.***
- ***My body is pure, clean and healthier from my detox fast.***
- ***I am now thinking constructively, not destructively!***

Instead of worrying about problems, she sought the answers in calm meditation. As she continued to rebuild her vitality, we introduced her to the complete Nerve Force Building Program detailed in this book. With a 24-hour fast each week and The Bragg Healthy Lifestyle diet, her physical problems soon faded away. She began taking her husband to the *AA – Alcoholics Anonymous* meetings, *(www.AA.org)* and this soon solved his drinking problem. This experience helped her as well. She realized the founders of AA had recognized the role of Nerve Force in helping to solve one of the major problems of our times – alcoholism! She also found it helped her, as it did other AA members at the opening of each meeting or during her own private meditations to recite and follow this world famous Sanskrit prayer:

Give me the Serenity to accept what cannot be changed;
the Courage to change what can be changed;
and the Wisdom to know the difference.

This woman also developed the Nerve Force necessary to cope with her two teenage children. She was now better equipped to communicate with them; something she had not been able to do for years. She found she could bridge the generation gap and find the essential common ground to meet and hold discussions with her children. Both of them made a big turn around, went on to college, got splendid grades and good jobs.

By changing personal behavior, we can reduce our risk of dying early by 70% to 80%. – John Graham, Former President, Professional Society for Risk Analysis • sra.org

---

Realize that everything connects to everything else. – Leonardo da Vinci

Keep Your Nerves Healthy and Strong

So someone who was ready to destroy herself got a new lease on life by turning to Natural Living and simply following the Laws of Mother Nature. We were only guides to help her to help herself! That is what we want to do for you, the reader of this book! **We want to teach you how to build powerful Nerve Force by following the Eternal Laws of Mother Nature. Remember that life flows through your nerves. An alert and active nervous system is therefore the greatest gift of Mother Nature, for it is through the nerves that we experience the pleasures that make life wonderful and worth living.** To be dull-nerved means to be mentally and physically dull – insensitive to the higher phases of life, incapable of deep emotions such as love, and lacking the spark-force of character and life.

It is true that highly sensitive and active nerves – when abused – are a menace to health. But don't consider it a misfortune if you are born with "high-energy" nerves. Although this means you must be wise in words and actions, for you could "explode" if you don't use caution.

Two Sides of the Shield – Physical & Mental

The story is told of two knights who fought a duel to the death over the exact color of their King's shield which hung high above the center of his castle's great hall. One knight claimed that his sovereign's shield was red. The other asserted just as vehemently that it was green. After their tragic battle someone looked up at the shield – one side was green, the other side was red. Similarly there are two sides to the Shield of Health – the physical and the mental – both equally important!

It's sad to note for centuries the problem of health has been approached primarily on the physical level. Now we know we must do everything in our power not

Do what you can to improve, with what you have, where you are!
– Theodore Roosevelt, 26th American President, 1933–1945

Dear friend, I wish above all things that thou may prosper and be in health, even as the soul prospers. – 3 John 2

only to keep ourselves physically fit, but also to keep ourselves mentally fit! You will accomplish the first goal by following our Nerve Force Program and The Bragg Healthy Lifestyle. You'll address the second by practicing your daily meditations and prayer, during which you must examine your body – inner and outer self – using reason, logic and intelligence to seek and find the answers to solve your long-term and daily problems.

A Strong Mind in a Strong Body

These two states – the physical and mental – are so closely interrelated that it is impossible to separate them. Physical health affects mental alertness and mental control imposes the necessary discipline to maintain physical health. For perfect health – including powerful Nerve Force – we must have a strong mind in a strong body. Flesh does not operate through intelligence and reasoning, but through the five senses. Your body's first reaction in response to stimuli is to gratify the senses, such as satisfying hunger: for example, eating something that is pleasing to the taste, regardless of negative health benefits. **A vicious circle can evolve into an unhealthy body and mind. The devitalized popular foods in the Standard American Diet (S.A.D.) fail to supply proper nourishment! Flesh becomes weary, and Nerve Force becomes depleted on "foodless" fast junk foods.**

Instead of seeking help from Mother Nature's healthy foods, human flesh seeks quick gratification from the temporary, but false sense of well-being provided by coffee, tea, sugar, colas, pills, alcohol, and tobacco. This gratification is temporary relief only! It causes further energy depletion, which can lead to stronger drug use that can create the "false illusions" of feeling good.

Many people go through their life committing partial suicide. They destroy their health, youth, talents, energies and creative qualities. Indeed, to learn how to be good to oneself is often harder than to learn how to be good to others. – Joshua Liebman, Ph.D., American Rabbi, best-selling author "Peace of Mind"

Before speaking put it to this test: Is it kind? Is it good? Is it necessary? This Program is designed to help you control your nerves and build a powerful Nerve Force – and use it wisely!

Now, your reason and intelligence will tell you that unhealthy living is slow bodily suicide! **Since the brain is your body's "miracle captain" computer, reckless living causes mental deterioration! To build a strong body, the mind must be strong enough to assume control of the body, and establish and faithfully maintain The Bragg Healthy Lifestyle habits.** A beneficial cycle will then ensue, for a healthy body is your best insurance for a healthy mind and powerful, healthy Nerve Force!

A strong mind will generate positive thoughts and help to keep the body on the High Road to Health. However, the mind can also produce negative thoughts and suggestions, so your mind must be strong enough to resist these impulses. A properly functioning body should have a mechanical precision that protects it from negative mental interference. Our first duty, therefore, must be to educate our bodies to follow The Bragg Healthy Lifestyle. **As we improve the physical part of our human machinery, we will also improve our mental state. The brain demands five times as much blood as any other of our organs. Give it what it needs – healthy nutrition, exercise, deep breathing and by doing so faithfully – it will be grateful and perform better!**

Make Your Body Worry Proof

The Greeks created this perfect phrase for this human interrelationship: **A strong mind in a strong body.** No one said it better. If you're mentally upset, you can walk miles – but if physically sick, clear, constructive thinking is virtually impossible! By raising your physical health standards, your mental abilities will increase accordingly. **Be on good terms with your body to enjoy your mind fully.**

If our mental machinery is sluggish, we look to our physical machinery for explanations. What is the reason and the remedy for our halting thoughts and stumbling sentences? We usually find we need a break and some exercise. We refresh and recharge with a long, brisk walk, deeply breathing in the fresh air that cleans the cobwebs from our brains! When our mental creativity returns, then we return to our writing, the words flow effortlessly from our brains to the tips of our fingers – it's exciting. Dad and I have loved sharing our wisdom with you!

There Is No Reward For Worry

We have always believed that abnormal mental states have physical explanations. Cheerfulness may be the result of sunshine communicating a sense of well-being to the cortical area of the brain. Gardens, flowers, and nature scenes have calming effects on your nervous system. A harmonious interior design may soothe the mind through the five senses. Kaiser Hospital had rooms in pastel colors.

Smiling is a great example of the close interaction between the mental and the physical states. We smile naturally when we are feeling happy. Have you ever tried making yourself smile when you are feeling blue? Try it! Physical acts of smiling *(takes 13 muscles)* and also laughing nearly always trigger mental reactions that makes you feel better! Don't forget it requires mental effort in the first place to make you "smile away your tears!"

Let's make a strong pledge to use the necessary mental discipline it takes to establish and maintain the physical discipline making the body "worry proof" (impervious to negative thoughts)! This will help to keep our minds healthy and free from worry. Educate the brawn and train the brain! You will then attain the healthier ideal balance for both – perfect physical and mental health.

Help with Panic Attacks

Panic attack episodes are intense apprehension or fear that are of sudden, yet brief duration. The most common symptoms may include trembling, chest pain, nausea and hyperventilation. Vitamin B deficiency and an unhealthy lifestyle may be major causes! There are strategies that you can use to help stop the attack when you feel one coming on. 1) Deep breathing can reduce symptoms. 2) Recognize that it is just a panic attack and it is temporary and will pass. 3) Close your eyes. Too much stimuli can feed your panic attack. 4) Use muscle relaxation techniques. 5) Picture your happy place. 6) Keep lavender on hand – the scent is soothing (*healthline.com*).

The body and mind are so closely connected that not even a single word or thought can come into existence without being reflected in the personality and health of the individual. – John Holmes Prentiss, 1784-1861

Good Posture Promotes Healthier Nerves

Look at yourself in the mirror. Do your shoulders slump? Is your upper back round? Do you have a protruding potbelly? Are you a swayback? Can you see the reasons why your back has the right to ache? The bending, slumping, ligament-stretching and the force of gravity has taken its toll. If you are a backache sufferer due to weak muscles and bad posture, (see page 23) don't despair, you can restore back comfort with this simple posture exercise (see below), The Bragg Healthy Lifestyle and read *Bragg Back & Foot Fitness Program* Book (page 218).

It has often been said that backache is the penalty man must pay for the privilege of standing and walking upright on two feet, often wearing uncomfortable shoes. Every infant struggles to stand instinctively on his own two feet and walk. He need not be taught. He will attempt this bipedal gait even if left alone most of the time and never instructed. It is natural for a human being to stand and walk in this manner. This is interesting, because there are no animals which spend all of their standing and walking hours on two feet, not even gorillas or chimpanzees. These apes use their hands and arms to help them move about. The world's strongest gorilla would be unable to follow a busy person, walking erectly, for more than a short time. This is because human beings are meant to walk erect with good posture.

Bragg Posture Exercise Brings Miracles & Gives Instant Youthfulness – Do This Exercise Daily!

Stand (feet 8" apart) before a mirror and stretch up your spine. Tighten buttocks and suck in stomach muscles, lift up rib cage, put chest out, shoulders back, and chin up slightly. Line body up straight (nose plumbline straight to belly button), drop hands to sides and swing arms to normalize your posture. Do this posture exercise daily and miraculous changes will happen! You are retraining and strengthening your muscles to stand straight for health and youthfulness. Remember when you slump, you also cramp your precious machinery. This posture exercise (do 2-3 times daily) will retrain your frame to sit, stand and walk tall for health, fitness and longevity!

When your body is completely relaxed then you will experience an inner peace, inner serenity and the true joy of living.

WHERE DO YOU STAND?

POSTURE CHART

	PERFECT	FAIR	POOR
HEAD			
SHOULDERS			
SPINE			
HIPS			
ANKLES			
NECK			
UPPER BACK			
TRUNK			
ABDOMEN			
LOWER BACK			

Your posture carries you through life from your head to your feet. This is your human vehicle and you are truly a miracle! Cherish, respect and always protect it by living The Bragg Healthy Lifestyle. – Patricia Bragg

Good posture helps prevent backaches and related problems.

Remember – Your posture can make or break your health!

Start Building Your Nerve Force Today!

1. Put a stop to all undue nerve waste. Use prayer and meditation to clear mind of worries, fears, negative thoughts and emotions that drain away nerve energy. Replace these with clear statement of your goals. See the image of yourself as you want to become and with the confidence that you will achieve your purpose. Maintain a positive attitude that will greatly assist you in building powerful Nerve Force to gain your goals. See pages 47-62.

2. Get 8 hours of deep, restful sleep every night. Lower your stress levels and when possible take power naps and a short siesta after midday meal. See pages 63-76.

3. Adopt a program of eating that will keep you internally clean and healthy. Give up all devitalized foods, drinks and all artificial stimulants: tobacco, alcohol, cola drinks, coffee, tea, salt, refined sugars, and eat a preponderance of organic fruits and vegetables – both raw and lightly cooked. Fast 24 hours weekly taking only distilled water and the vinegar drink (recipe page 108). Take a 7-to 10-day fast yearly to help unburden your nerves of all toxic poisons, obstructions and build-ups of any kind. See pages 77-110.

4. Have a daily exercise program. Get out in fresh air and exercise to improve circulation and sleep better. Walk briskly, jog, jump rope, swim, dance, do tai chi, Qi gong and play games. Keep your 640 body muscles active and healthy! Buy a pedometer (*www.fitbit.com*) – fun to monitor walks, runs, etc. See pages 111-122.

5. Breathe deeply. Get more life-giving oxygen deep down in the lower lungs. Oxygen is your greatest "Nerve Tonic." Nerve Force is built with oxygen. The raw fruits and vegetables in your diet are loaded with oxygen, and taking purifying fasts will increase your body's capacity for absorbing oxygen. Through deep breathing you help cleanse your blood of toxic carbon dioxide and fill it with vital oxygen, which is needed and taken to every cell in your body! See pages 123-132.

I am going to obey the Wise Laws of God and Mother Nature. I know I will find more health, peace of mind, joy and serenity.

6. Bathe daily. Drench your body with hot and cold water to increase your circulation, then enjoy healing rays of gentle sunlight. See pages 133-142.

7. Keep your emotions under control. Do not subject your nerves to stress that can be avoided. It is difficult enough to face and overcome the trials that you cannot avoid without going forth to seek other means of exhausting your nerves! See 143-152.

8. Relax your nerves. The natural rhythm of life is tension, then relaxation – like the beat of your heart. Strive to make your nervous system so powerful and healthy that your body will automatically shift from tension to relaxation. See pages 153-158.

9. Enjoy life. Don't forget to play and have fun as life goes on! That is one of the reasons you are here on earth – to enjoy it. Success and material possessions are all right in their place, but you must enjoy life each day to the fullest. Whistle, hum, sing, laugh and dance! Please keep away from dispensers of gloom. This old world has been a madhouse since it first began. **Do everything you can to make it a healthier, safer world and help improve yourself, family and friends and then others.** See pages 159-160.

Morning Resolve To Start Your Day

I will this day live a simple, sincere and serene life; repelling promptly every thought of impurity, discontent, anxiety, discouragement and fear. I will cultivate health, cheerfulness, happiness, charity and the love of brotherhood; exercising economy in expenditure, generosity in giving, carefulness in conversation and diligence in appointed service. In particular, I will be faithful in those habits of prayer, study, work, nutrition, physical exercise, deep breathing and good posture. I shall fast for a 24-hour period each week, eat only healthy foods and get sufficient sleep each night. I will make every effort to improve myself physically, mentally, emotionally and spiritually every day.

Morning Prayer used by Paul C. Bragg and Patricia Bragg

Gloom and bleakness steals joy, energy and color from your world. You can't save your life if you don't value it! – "Heart Healthy Living Magazine"

Open your mind, for the doors of wisdom are never shut. – Benjamin Franklin

YOUR STRESS SCALE TEST

Take This Quick Stress Quiz:

Indicate how strongly you agree with each of the following statements on a scale from 0 to 3:

0 = never 1 = sometimes 2 = often 3 = always

__ I have trouble relaxing.
__ I get frustrated when people are incompetent.
__ I feel tense and rushed.
__ I worry about work and other problems.
__ I have difficulty falling asleep.
__ I feel grief or loss.
__ I am exhausted by daily demands at work & home.
__ I feel stuck in a rat race.
__ No matter how hard I try, I never feel caught up.
__ I feel burdened by financial obligations.
__ I am under strain at work.
__ I feel lonely and unloved.
__ I am embarrassed to ask for assistance.
__ I feel overwhelmed by my responsibilities.
__ I can't stand criticism.
__ I'm afraid I'll lose my job or livelihood.
__ People let me down.
__ No matter what I achieve, I feel dissatisfied.
__ I stew in my anger rather than express it.
__ I feel apprehensive about the future.
__ My stress is caused by forces beyond my control.
__ I feel pressured by my commitments.
__ I have difficulty delegating.
__ I feel like running away.
__ My mind is churning and too busy.

_____ Total Score

- 0 to 18 = you are resilient and feel in charge of your life
- 19 to 37 = mild stress; with apprehension and some struggle
- 38 to 56 = moderate stress; feeling trapped, out of control
- 57 to 75 = high stress; life feels like one crisis after another

The Importance of NERVE FORCE

Nerve Depletion: A Lack of Nerve Energy

As previously noted, the millions of nerve cells that make up the vast Nervous System can be seen as reservoirs of nerve energy. The amount of nerve energy we store represents our entire precious Nerve Capital.

It is evident that if our nerve reservoirs are but 50% full of nerve energy – that is, half depleted – our nerve pressure will be half of what it should be. Thus our vital organs and muscles will receive only a fraction of the supply of Nerve Force necessary to enable them to perform their full duty, which is running the entire body.

Our nerve pressure is at its greatest height when our nerve cells are full of stored energy. We are then fully alive with physical and mental energy. No task seems too great, no strain too severe. We crave ways of letting off steam. That's when you become a human dynamo. You have double the energy and vitality of the average person! You have so much Nerve Force in your reservoir you are absolutely tireless! This is what my father and I have been able to attain for ourselves – and we want the same for you and for everyone! It's to be treasured and guarded.

As mentioned earlier, my father had been through the experience of extreme nerve depletion. There is no part of exhaustion that we cannot understand. Depletion and abuse of the nervous system leads to a motley group of organic, mental and physical weaknesses and disorders. The proper functioning of every muscle and every organ – in fact, every cell of the human body – depends directly upon the nerves for the initial impulse of life and power. It's inevitable that nerve depletion generally weakens the body and disturbs its proper functions – causing upsets.

Nerve Force is the basis for success...it is the dominant power of our existence.

It is not inevitable, however, that your Nerve Force must remain depleted. You can rebuild it! You don't have to drag yourself around fatigued and only half-alive! **Mother Nature intended you to be full of vitality and positive energy – regardless of your age! Follow The Bragg Healthy Lifestyle presented in this book and you will fill and maintain your reservoir with dynamic Nerve Force!**

Nerve Depression: Decreased Energy Flow

Nerve Depression means the shutting off of the nerve flow from the reservoirs, just as you would stop the water flow in a garden hose by stepping on it. No matter how full of energy your nerve reservoirs may be, your vital organs may be prevented from getting their normal supply of Nerve Force because of Nerve Depression.

The difference between Nerve Depletion and Nerve Depression is that the former can be a deep-seated general Nervous System weakness, whereas any Nerve Depression may be of a temporary nature. For instance, worry and grief can cause extreme Nerve Depression, which may result in death within a short time. The expression "died of a broken heart" can literally be true, because in some cases the heart is actually paralyzed by emotional distress! Nerve Depression has a direct and powerful paralyzing effect upon all the vital organs. A person who claims to be "worried to death" may be uttering a fatal truth!

Yet, we all have to face worries at times in our lives. You can't escape them. If you have the physical and mental nervous energy required, you can face almost any worry without letting it harm and tear you apart! A full reservoir of Nerve Force lets you take worries in stride!

Our best preparation for tomorrow is the proper use of today!

I know the sunny side of life. My Nerve Force gives me the power to radiate sunshine in the gloomiest of times. – Paul C. Bragg, N.D., Ph.D.

Of all the knowledge, the most worth having is the knowledge about health! The first requisite of a good life is to be a healthy person. – Herbert Spencer

Nerve Tension: Excessive Nervous Energy

Nerve Tension, stress and strain are caused by undue nervous excitement which produces over-activity of the nervous system, such as great fear and anger. It can even cause instant death. During the Great Depression of the early 1930s, Dad personally saw businessmen die from the tension, stress and strain of being financially ruined.

Under high Nerve Tension, a large volume of Nerve Force is poured out in a short space of time, thus causing extreme agitation of the vital organs. We have all observed that when we are angry or frightened our heart beats wildly, we breathe rapidly and our abdominal organs are topsy-turvy, sometimes causing sudden evacuation of the bowels or even some vomiting and the shakes.

Recognizing and Avoiding Hypertension

American Medical Association research indicates that people who have uncontrolled hypertension (high blood pressure) are more likely to develop coronary heart disease. They are six times more likely to develop congestive heart failure, and seven times more likely to have a stroke.

In the important Framingham Heart Study, doctors found hypertension responsible for 40% of congestive heart failure in men, and 60% in women. Hypertension was diagnosed in 91% of participants with congestive heart failure. The risk of developing congestive heart failure was twice as high in men, and three times as high in women, whose blood pressure was higher than normal (120/70) levels. Less than one quarter of the men and less than one third of the women lived more than 5 years after being diagnosed with congestive heart failure. **See website: *www.FraminghamHeartStudy.org***

Your blood vessels can be severely damaged by high blood pressure. The force of blood pushing hard through your arteries can shear and tear off cells from the inside lining; this leads to a build up of bulging plaque, made of fat, cholesterol and dead cells. Those with elevated blood cholesterol levels – especially "bad cholesterol" (low density lipoprotein, LDL) are at greater heart risk for developing fatty plaques. **(See Healthy Heart Habits, page 122.)**

Hypertension accelerates the process, and the plaques can grow and eventually block the passage of blood – known as atherosclerosis – which can even begin as early as childhood! Like hypertension, atherosclerosis is silent until there has been enough damage done to cause symptoms. Nearly 1 in 5 with silent atherosclerosis have a heart attack as their initial symptom.*

High blood pressure can also speed up the hardening of the arteries – arteriosclerosis. This occurs when the muscles in your blood vessels become thickened and hard, which narrows the arteries and makes them less flexible. Therefore, less blood passes through the vessels to the tissues, resulting in coronary artery disease.

An EKG – electrocardiogram – can determine whether your heart is damaged or enlarged. An EKG monitors your heart's electrical activity. Your doctor may also recommend an echocardiogram, to evaluate and see the size of your heart and how well it is functioning.

Not surprisingly, physically active people are much less apt to have high blood pressure than sedentary "couch potatoes." Your diet can also affect your blood pressure. Eating low or nonfat foods, fresh fruits and vegetables and whole-grain foods, can help lower your blood pressure. Eating excessive amounts of saturated fat will raise the level of cholesterol in your blood. This can lead to increased chances of heart disease as well as developing cancer, diabetes and other illnesses.

Calculating cholesterol and fat is unnecessary – just avoid animal foods which are the main source of harmful cholesterol (LDL). It's best to avoid foods that had a face. The "good" cholesterol (HDL) high density lipoprotein, is formed only in your body. The HDL cholesterol is a larger particle that helps to remove fat from the blood and the artery walls. **The Bragg Healthy Lifestyle with energy powered organic fruits, vegetables, whole grains, etc, a diet low in saturated fats, and getting plenty of exercise will help you avoid heart disease, hypertension and other life-threatening illnesses.**

Read the Bragg Healthy Heart Book to build a strong heart and prevent heart disease, strokes and heart attacks – the #1 killer of Americans.

High Blood Pressure in Adolescence

Childhood obesity is particularly troubling because the extra pounds often start kids on the path to health problems that were once confined to adults, such as high blood pressure, diabetes, and high cholesterol. This research strongly suggests overweight prevention may need to begin even before the first day of school, promoting good nutrition, as well as exercise and fitness.

In the last two decades, the prevalence of overweight children ages 6-11 has doubled and tripled for American teenagers. The annual National Health and Nutrition Examination Survey done by the Center for Disease Control and Prevention found that about 20-25% of U.S. children are overweight or at risk of becoming overweight.

According to the Mayo Clinic the incidence of childhood obesity is rapidly rising throughout the world. It is especially evident in the U.S. where many children live sedentary lives with too much time spent watching television or playing video games and eating more convenience fast foods, junk foods and sweets, which are typically higher in fat calories and low in healthy nutritional values. See web: *MayoClinic.com*.

Lower Your Blood Pressure Naturally

A government-sponsored Joint National Committee on Detection, Evaluation and Treatment of High Blood Pressure has been calling for a healthy (non-drug) lifestyle as a treatment for individuals with various forms of hypertension. Sadly over a third of Americans (1 in 3) have high blood pressure or hypertension.

News on High Blood Pressure and Diet

Researchers from New York Presbyterian Hospital have found that the mineral components of diets can significantly lower blood pressure, especially if one is suffering from hypertension. The specific minerals were potassium, magnesium and calcium. Eating a low-fat diet aids in lowering high blood pressure and cholesterol levels.

The role of the mind and emotions in our state of health is a vital one. By understanding this relationship we can play a greater role in our wellbeing.
– Mark Hyman, M.D., Huffpost Healthy Living • HuffingtonPost.com

Researchers examined 400 airport traffic controllers, who work under stressful high-pressure conditions. After a three year period, the air traffic controllers developed hypertension at a rate of three to four times higher than the normal population. Other research indicated individuals who move from rural towns to the big city, have an increase of blood pressure. **Stress can result in significant elevations in blood pressure; this can overwhelm your cardiovascular system and make you a prime heart attack, stroke and illness candidate.**

More than two decades of research in biofeedback have demonstrated that we can bring many Autonomic Nervous System (ANS) (see page 2) functions under our control if information about how to do so is made available. As we practice and identify what we're doing, figuring out what works and what doesn't, we learn to improve our skills – like learning to drive a car. Obtaining biofeedback (that monitors your heart rate and skin temperature) can aid in developing sensitivity and the ability to modify your internal physiology towards better health.

Dr. Barbara Brown in her book *Stress and the Art of Biofeedback* states, "When the mind receives information about itself, its body, how it reacts to stress and how it can return to well-being, mental faculties of awareness and understanding are then roused to action! By some obscure capacity, cognitive faculties are set in motion to restore the mind and body to a state of balance and relieve the effects of stress." By learning correct breathing techniques (read *Bragg Super Power Breathing* Book, page 217), and muscular relaxation and imagery, the mind learns a new mental and emotional response! This eventually will result in modifications of the vital hypothalamus and limbic system – a specialized area within the subcortical brain, often referred to as the emotional brain. With practice, you can establish the voluntary control of the unconscious process and bridge the gap between the conscious and the unconscious.

A study found that young adults (ages 18-30) with healthy blood pressure go on to have better thinking and memory skills in mid-life than their peers with higher blood pressure. Higher blood pressure readings early in life were associated with poor performance on memory, learning and decision processing speed.

Biofeedback Empowers You to Relax

A controlled study by Dr. Keith Sedlacek divided hypertensive patients into two groups. One group learned simple relaxation techniques accompanied by a bio-feedback method; the other received only medication. **After a four month period, blood pressure had decreased in the relaxation/biofeedback group from an average of 144/95 to 120/70. Visit biofeedback website: *www.Brain-Trainer.com.*** In contrast, the medication-only group showed no significant decline in blood pressure over the four months. These antihypertensive drugs are not only costly, but often have unpleasant side effects which may increase the risk of cardiovascular disease! Therefore, a "step zero" approach is recommended – medication is gradually reduced, then eliminated to "zero" for the individuals who can regain control of their blood pressure through non-pharmacological, healthy lifestyle methods!

CIP – Constant Instant Practice is a process that rapidly re-establishes equilibrium in just a few moments and helps break the stress cycle naturally at its source.

This CIP includes 3 steps: • deepening your breathing • relaxing your muscles • warming your hands and feet

The instant you detect stress, extend and deepen your breath – for uninterrupted, smooth, deep breathing *(your invisible staff of life)* is the key to stress control. Relaxing muscles, especially around the shoulders, back and jaw counters the body's tendency to tighten under stress! Warming the hands and feet will decrease sympathetic nervous system activity. Your hands and feet play a critical role in your response to stress! While your body temperature varies no more than a few degrees from 98.6°, the temperature of hands and feet can vary nearly 25 degrees. If you're calm and relaxed, hands and feet will become warmer. Warming your hands and feet (in hot vinegar water) calms nerves and helps increase circulation that also helps normalize the blood pressure!

Prevention is always wisest and preferable to the cure!

Breathing is our miracle connection to life, through the body and heart, leading us to a healthy wholeness of being and giving us spirit for living life to its fullest. – S. Hainer, M.S.

Self-Pity is a Nerve and Energy Robber

Another demon that you must dissipate is self-pity. Feeling sorry for yourself is a complete waste of energy. It blocks sympathy and help from others! When sorrow comes your way – face it and know that time will bring relief. Never accept despair or defeat! **Remember that it is never too late to give yourself a second chance!**

Even if your past was a very happy one, don't try to live in it. Life does not run backward! Energy – a principle of Mother Nature – only moves forward! We cannot use it for ourselves in any way that is contrary to its laws. We cannot expect to hold energy, which moves forward, if we are thinking backward. **Our energy depends upon our Nerve Force. That's why we must build powerful Nerve Force that will enable us to daily create health and happiness in all phases of life!**

Self-Talk and Even Write to Yourself: You Can Be Your Best Health Therapist!

Kenneth Pelletier, Ph.D., an authority on stress, states that individuals who manage stress well – and even thrive on it – have learned to create "regular islands of peace" in their daily lives. You can achieve this by regularly taking brief moments of relaxation that brings your body and mind back to a state of homeostasis (or peaceful balance), as well as using CIP method page 33.

Constructive Self-Talk and Mental Rehearsal can also help you to manage stress more effectively – for example, developing statements to say to yourself during times of stress. This internal dialogue along with the CIP method will assist you in getting your body and mind into balance.

Take time to do something healthy for yourself.
Improving your outlook on life goes a long way in improving health.
Take care of yourself naturally and positively.
– Bragg Friend, Dr. Bob Martin, "Secret Nerve Cures"

Negative thoughts influence our health!
Studies show negative brain activity could be linked to a weakened immune system. – MayoClinic.com.

POSITIVE HEALTH STATEMENTS TO USE:

- I listen to my inner self – I can accomplish miracles!
- Feeling stressed is not going to help this situation.
- I'll just get started and then I'll be all right.
- Take things one step at a time, then everything will go smoother and happier. Smile more!
- Relax, be calm, plan, plot, and follow through.
- Problems are an opportunity to engage in solutions.
- I've done this before and I can do it again! Smile!
- Just take it easy . . . remember one step at a time.
- Try to think, hear or see things from other person's point of view. Relax, breathe deep and slow!
- The harder things get, the more dedicated I am.
- It takes two to have a conflict. I'm not going to participate in something that's not important and that will put more unwanted stress on me!

Create some of your own constructive, positive stress-management phrases. Write them on an index card and tape up in your home, office and car. Make them part of your everyday positive thought process. Mentally rehearse – see, hear and feel yourself successfully responding to and managing any stressful situation which may arise! You can create new neurogenic circuits for healthier behavior patterns by imagining positive ways you wish to handle any future stressful circumstances!

Maximize Benefits of Positive Affirmations

Your happiness and your success in life is determined by the thoughts you hold. By consistently repeating positive affirmations you reinforce the new positive inner image you have of yourself. Let yourself really feel them. To maximize the benefits – use positive affirmations every day for at least 30 days. Also stop thinking negatively and replace with your favorite positive affirmations. For more positive affirmations see : *www.VitalAffirmations.com*

Some of life's greatest pleasures happen when we slow down, and start enjoying the little things that brighten our life. – MacAnderson.com

---

I give thanks daily for all the Miracle Blessings I receive.
– Patricia Bragg

Some Need Professional Help

If you are frequently irritated, angry, anxious, severely depressed, bitter or burned out and are unable to resolve your problems, it may be advisable to work with a competent therapist. You might have to interview a few to find the right match. Call several and say you **are seeking a therapist – could you drop in and say hello – then look, talk and feel if it's the right therapist. Lots of people are smart to have wise advisers to converse with, and work out the roller coaster problems they often face.**

Nerve Force is Powerful and So Important

Nervous tension, stress and strain can cause an excessive expenditure of Nerve Force. That is why we feel "drained" after a sudden fright, upset or great anger. Under these conditions even people whose nerve reservoirs are depleted to the lowest level can – for a short period – pour out an enormous quantity of nerve energy that produces unusual strength and adrenaline. For example, someone who is involved in an accident or emergency.

We once read a newspaper account of two young boys, both only 14 years old, who were hiking in the forest when suddenly a thunder storm appeared. Lightning struck a tree which fell on one of the boys, pinning him down. He screamed in pain and fright. The other boy – exerting superhuman strength granted by his Nerve Force – lifted the heavy tree off his friend, put him on his back and ran for 5 miles to get help. The next day, the injured boys parents and several men went to the accident scene. Four adult men could not lift the tree! *A miracle for sure!*

We do not want to wait for such an emergency to drain our vital powerful Nerve Force from our reservoirs or to prove that we can exert it. We want to develop powerful Nerve Force that will keep our reservoirs full, and be aware of the fact that we have it when needed!

God promises miracle healings to people who fast and pray.

Develop healthy self-esteem to generate positive lifestyle habits that promote more serenity, peace and love in your life. – Patricia Bragg

Physical and Mental Deterioration

When your Nerve Force becomes depleted, you feel mentally and physically fatigued and exert yourself only by the utmost stimulation of your will power. In doing this you put draining stress, strain and tension upon yourself. It's then you try to fight your fatigue with unhealthy stimulants such as coffee, "Pep Pills," alcohol or drugs that sadly will further exhaust your nerves as you head towards a complete nervous breakdown!

It's then that we begin to feel ourselves getting old, although we may still be young. A more pronounced decline is seen in our physical, mental and organic forces as our Nerve Force becomes more depleted! We lose our sex drive and the sparkle fades from our eyes. We lose the spring in our step and we lose our skin and muscle tone. Because of the sluggishness of our vital organs, we may begin to excessively gain or lose weight.

Impaired Metabolism Causes Body Imbalance

Nerve exhaustion seriously impairs a basic process of the body known as the Metabolism. This is the process by which nutritive material is transformed into living tissue (constructive), or living tissue and nutrients are broken down (destructive) and used to produce energy. **Every cell in the body is constantly engaged in either the constructive or destructive process, and every vital organ is a part of the intricate machinery of Metabolism. It's the life process, the basis of all health and all vital power.**

When nerves are normal, there's a balanced harmony between the constructive and destructive processes of Metabolism. When this precious Nerve Force is depleted or exhausted the natural, healthy equilibrium is thrown off balance and the most noticeable results are excessive loss or gain of weight and lack of energy! (See page 165-166.)

A healthy diet, therefore, cannot be gauged in mere calories. We must eat healthy foods that will help build our Nerve Force! This way there will be sufficient nerve energy to convert the food into tissue and then into energy to maintain a healthy balanced metabolism.

Post-Traumatic Stress Disorder – "PTSD"

According to the National Institute of Mental Health (NIMH) nearly 7.7 million Americans have PTSD at any given time. Although more men than women undergo "traumatic" events in their lifetime, more women develop PTSD. The symptoms of PTSD can range from mild to life-changing; from concerns to major depressive or panic disorders that can shatter a person's well-being and health. This can lead to intense phobias, paralyzing fear or feelings of helplessness and horror. Maintaining good physical health is a key to recovery.

Nervous Disorders Upset the Stomach

As stated before, the Sympathetic Nervous System governs the vital organs. The master branch of this system is referred to as the Pneumo-Gastric Nerve System, whose center is the solar plexus, or "abdominal brain," known in Yoga as our wise second brain. **The pneumo-gastric nerve governs breathing and digestion, hence its name – pneumo (lung) and gastric (stomach). It is closely allied with the functioning of all the organs.**

Sometimes even the slightest nervous upheaval can affect the pneumogastric nerve. We have all observed an uneasy feeling in the stomach when we worry, our solar plexus is affected, and sometimes the back. In cases of severe Nerve Strain, the stomach may rebel against your putting food in by throwing it up. When upset don't eat.

Millions Suffer From Nervous Indigestion

Nearly every form of indigestion, gastric and other abdominal troubles may be traced almost directly to a nervous disturbance or an abnormal condition of the pneumogastric nerve. This applies especially to the conditions usually grouped under "Nervous Indigestion." These are often too casually dismissed by most as temporary discomfort to be relieved by a quick drugstore remedy which merely postpones the future inevitable!

The indigestion conditions include fermentation, gas, heartburn, sour stomach, hyperacidity and stomach bloating, which often result in shortness of breath and pressure on the heart. These conditions can produce heart irregularity, palpitations and even heart failure.

Heartburn = Higher Risk for Cancer

According to a report in the *New England Journal of Medicine,* those with daily heartburn or indigestion have a higher risk of esophageal cancer, especially those who smoke, drink alcohol or caffeine and consume fatty foods and chocolate. The acid levels in your stomach soar, eventually causing an alteration of esophageal cells which can become malignant.

University of Tennessee Researcher, Glenn Eisen, has cited recent studies indicating that heartburn or indigestion, clinically known as gastroesophageal reflux disease (GERD) – stomach acid which bubbles up into the esophagus – can be treated with diet and lifestyle changes. "If you need any acid-reducing drugs more than once a week, you should see your doctor."

Frequent dilation and bloating of the stomach, due to gas formation very often leads to permanent dilation and the forming of "pockets" from which your food cannot drain. In these pockets a very serious condition – ulceration of the stomach – may begin. A prominent surgeon told us that many serious stomach disorders are the result of this stomach ulceration.

It is very evident that we should combat the first indication of Nervous Indigestion with the means at our command, and not seek fast, temporary relief. We must get at the cause and correct it! There are no shortcuts to health! You must earn your health and Nerve Force.

Depression and Stress May Affect Diabetics and Cause Heart Attacks

According to Reuters Health Publication, a study has found that people with insulin-dependent diabetes who reported feeling depressed, anxious, or stressed out were among the least likely to successfully lower their blood sugar levels. The study found that persons with diabetes have the potential to benefit from realization-based therapies such as biofeedback, meditation and prayer.

Diabetes affects 34 million Americans and is classified into two types: Type 1 and type 2 which affects 90-95% of cases. It's a major underlying cause of cardiovascular and kidney disease.

Another study done by the National Institute on Ageing in Bethesda, MD, has found that when older men get depressed, heart attacks aren't far behind. They studied 3,701 people over 70 years of age, for six years. Among women, depression did not increase the risk for heart attack or angina. However, among the men, the risk for heart attack or angina was almost double. When men are diagnosed with depression, it's important that they be closely evaluated for cardiovascular disease.

Other studies have shown that women are twice as likely as men to be diagnosed with clinical depression. According to researchers, the daily strains of work in and out of the home, coupled with feeling unappreciated by their partners and family, cause women to regularly think about their feelings. In turn, these thoughts feed stress. Women can help themselves by gaining greater control and solving their life problems, rather than dwelling on them. Also more education, achieving higher-level jobs and improving and enjoying work and home life are wise steps.

Nerve Depletion Promotes Constipation

Nerve depletion robs health and energy and promotes constipation. The action of the bowels depends as much upon nerve stimulation as the heart and lungs do. The bowels of a chronically constipated person will move freely when their nerves receive a violent shock, such as sudden fright, bad news or a violent emotional upset.

Refined foods and the like increase constipation. In order to be entirely free of sluggish bowels, your food must contain fiber, moisture and lubrication. These important elements are found in organic raw fruits and coarse vegetables, such as celery, beets, broccoli, cabbage and carrots, etc.

Many people will tell you they cannot eat raw fruits and vegetables. This is because the Nerve Force in their stomach and intestines is at a low ebb and they don't have enough nervous energy to digest such foods. In fact, people on a bland diet often don't have the nervous energy to digest even the softest foods! That is the reason why so many people are nervous wrecks! They cannot digest any food, and therefore the nervous system, as well as the rest of the body suffers from malnutrition. We've met people who look like scarecrows, who are so low in Nerve Force that its as if they are literally starving to death!

For Easier-Flowing Bowel Movements:

It's natural to squat to have bowel movements. It opens up the anal area more directly. When on the toilet, putting feet up 6-8" on a waste basket or footstool gives the same squatting effect. Now raise and stretch your hands above your head so the transverse colon can empty completely with ease. It's vital to drink eight glasses of water daily! (pages 101 and 122)

Feed Your Nerves – Don't Destroy Them!

Digestive and stomach trouble in extremely nervous people leads to a cycle of evils. First, nerve depletion impairs the power of the digestive organs. This creates toxic poisons which attack and further deplete the nerves. When nerve tissue is burned by toxic poisons, the nervous system can't function properly. Every victim that has indigestion problems, especially nervous indigestion, has observed that their nerves and health suffer correspondingly to the severity of the attack of indigestion. Few realize the beginning of the trouble lies in the weakness of their nerves (nerve exhaustion).

Avoid Junk Foods and Harmful Stimulants That Cause Nerve Burnout & Health Problems

People with impaired nerves should use the greatest care in food selections. Foods that continually cause indigestion should be avoided. Many people who drink coffee, for example, will suffer from indigestion afterwards. The same is often true of rich white flour and sugar pastries, ice cream, candy, cake, cookies, potato chips, hot dogs, greasy foods, hamburgers, ham, bacon, luncheon meats, catsup, and so many other devitalized foods. Many people also have severe stomach upsets from drinking alcoholic beverages.

ELIMINATE THE "DRIBBLES" EXERCISE:

To keep the bladder and sphincter muscles toned and tightened, urinate – stop – urinate – stop, 4 to 6 times, twice daily when voiding, especially after the age of 40. This simple exercise works wonders for men and women.

Tobacco, alcohol and caffeine drinks like coffee, tea *(many with caffeine)*, and colas are brutal whips that goad nerves into action. Unfortunately, the nerves don't have energy to obey for long. The drug caffeine stimulates the Central Nervous System and the coffee drinker gets a "lift" when caffeine activates the nervous energy from the reserves. In time, this brings on nerve depletion and causes serious troubles within the Nervous System.

According to an analysis made by the Council on Pharmacy of the American Medical Association, an average cup of coffee contains about 150 mg. of caffeine. When you drink 6 cups of coffee a day, your system assimilates almost 1 gram of toxic caffeine!

Your Gut Influences Your Emotional Health

It is estimated that millions of Americans suffer from some type of depressive disorder. Medications for such disorders may cause you to experience more serious problems in the long run. Not many people are aware that your digestive health is an important factor in your mental and emotional health. Studies suggest that poor gastrointestinal inflammation may be the culprit for emotional disorders. Dr. Mercola (*mercola.com*) explains that this actually makes perfect sense when you take note of the intricate connection between your brain and your gut. He says that your gut has the ability to impact your mind, mood, heart, and behavior, as it contains high concentrations of serotonin, a hormone that is linked to mood regulation.

Your gut is home to trillions of micro-organisms or "good bacteria" that influence numerous functions in your body, including your mood. By eating a diet rich in processed foods, sweetened beverages, or any sugar-laden product, the balance of good and bad bacteria in your digestive tract can be compromised; excessive sugar allows harmful bacteria to thrive! Sugar consumption also triggers chemical reactions in your body that promote chronic inflammation; excessive insulin release can result in hypoglycemia – which may trigger depression as well as agitation, anger, anxiety, panic attacks, and even an increased suicide risk.

According to one study, depression is often diagnosed alongside gut inflammation and auto-immune diseases; as well as cardiovascular problems, neurodegenerative disorders, Type 2 Diabetes and cancer, which are all related to chronic low-grade inflammation.

To optimize your gut flora, Dr. Mercola recommends:

- **Increase consumption of fermented foods.** Try pickled fermentations of cabbage (sauerkraut), turnips, eggplants, cucumbers squash and carrots. Also kefir (organic grass-fed milk), natto, and kimchi.
- **Take a probiotic supplement.**

Living The Bragg Healthy Lifestyle May Reverse Cellular Ageing!

In a recent study in *The Lancet Oncology Journal*, research has shown that healthy lifestyle changes can have an impact on ageing and age-related diseases on a cellular level – by increasing the length of telomeres. Telomeres are the "caps" that protect the ends of the chromosomes; similar to plastic caps on the end of shoelaces to stop them from fraying. Shorter telomeres have been linked with cell ageing and the increased risk of age-related diseases like cancer, dementia, and premature death.

Acclaimed Health Researcher, Dr. Dean Ornish, has conducted research on the effects of lifestyle changes on coronary heart disease for years. In this study, Dr. Ornish assigned 35 men, with low-risk prostate cancer, who were not being treated for their cancers but being monitored. They were split into two groups, one group of 10 men were assigned to make lifestyle

High Salty Foods May Cause Cellular Ageing

According to a study from the Medical College of Georgia, lowering sodium intake, especially if overweight or obese, may slow down the cellular ageing process that plays an important role in the development of heart disease. The study examined the effect of a high salt diet on the length of telomeres – the protective ends on chromosomes. They found that telomeres were much shorter in overweight and obese teens with high salt intake, but not in normal weight teens with high salt intake. The study does suggest that high sodium intake impacts telomeres shortening process.

changes – including eating a plant-based, vegan diet of whole foods, exercising moderately, meditation and yoga – for five years; while the other group did not make any lifestyle changes at all. The study found that healthy telomere length actually increased among the men assigned to the positive lifestyle changes. Meanwhile, telomere length decreased among the other men not assigned to any lifestyle changes! **Dr. Ornish summed up the research, *"To the extent we are willing to make changes to our diet and lifestyle, we can change things that were once thought to be impossible."*** For further info see web: *ornish.com.*

Millions Suffer From Nerve Exhaustion

How often do you hear of people going from doctor to doctor seeking relief for some mysterious malady or because "something's the matter" with them? Although repeated examinations fail to show that any organ is diseased or especially weak, these people persist seeking. The usual verdict of the physician is, *"There's nothing the matter with you, except you're a little run-down. You should go away and have a good rest."* In nearly every case, the real cause of this run-down unhealthy, toxic condition is Nerve Exhaustion, a very serious health problem!

In this age of strenuous living, the nerves are taxed so greatly that nearly everyone is a victim of some Nerve Exhaustion to a degree. The higher the state of mental faculties, the greater danger of nerve depletion. That's the reason why there are over 63.3 million people with mental disorders as their primary diagnosis in hospitals and physician's offices yearly in the U.S. (*cdc.gov*). There's also an increasing numbers of uncontrollable and mentally challenged children who present grave problems to their parents and educators in our country.

CORONARY DYSFUNCTION IN WOMEN WITH STRESS:
Researchers found that emotional stressors such as those provoking anger, may cause changes in the nervous system that controls heart rate and triggers a type of coronary artery dysfunction that occurs more frequently in women than men.

Get organized, be self-disciplined to live a healthy, long, fulfilled life.

There are many forms of nervousness. Each should be considered a warning sign to get busy at once, to build and restore the depleted Nerve Force. Moodiness is just one form of nervousness. Being "all keyed up" and unable to stop talking is another. Some people feel "all tied up." Others develop super-sensitive reactions, crying and going into emotional tantrums over the smallest matters. There are also those who become argumentative and aggressive, ready to fight and quarrel for no reason.

There is a long list of nervous conditions such as an upset, nervous stomach and headaches, sharp pains under the heart, heart palpitations and trembling cold hands and fingers. Some people lose interest in life and in everything and just sit around and brood. Others are overcome by waves of panic! They feel that something terrible is going to happen to them or one of their loved ones. Many people are overwhelmed by fears of all kinds (see more on fears on pages 55-62).

Remember Life Flows Through Your Nerves and that you alone have the power to generate the needed Nerve Force which is going to flow through your nerves. But you must work and earn it! It won't be handed to you on a silver platter. You must earn the good things of life. Everything in life has a price tag. What you put into this Nerve Force Building Program is what you will reap from it – no more, no less – it's all up to you!

There is absolutely nothing complicated about this Program we have outlined for you in this book. It's a simple, natural healthy lifestyle. Follow it – you can become a human dynamo regardless of your age.

Our Personal Health Message to You

You can become a powerhouse of dynamic energy, strength and vitality. You can build an inexhaustible reservoir of powerful Nerve Force. Nothing can stop you except yourself!

Love, kindness and compassion are necessities, not luxuries . . . without them humanity cannot survive. – The Dalai Lama

Through our actions and deeds, rather than promises, let us display the essence of love – perfect harmony in motion! – Philip Glyn, Welsh Poet

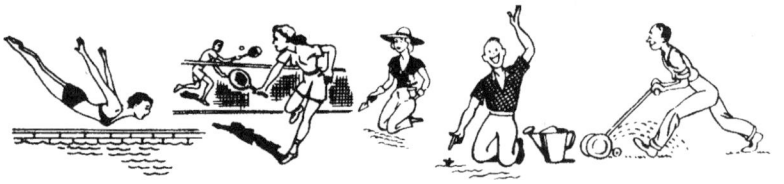

Live The Bragg Healthy Lifestyle To Enjoy a Lifetime of Super Health!

In a broad sense, *"The Bragg Healthy Lifestyle for the Total Person"* is a combination of physical, mental, emotional, social and spiritual components. The ability of the individual to function effectively in their environment depends on how smoothly these components function as a whole. Of all the qualities that comprise an integrated personality, a totally healthy, fit body is one of the most desirable . . . so start today on your goals for more health, happiness and peace in your life!

A person is said to be totally physically fit if they function as a total personality with efficiency and without pain or discomfort. This is to have a painless, tireless, and ageless body. You possess sufficient muscular strength and endurance to maintain a healthy posture. You can successfully carry on the duties imposed by life and the environment, and meet any emergencies satisfactorily and have enough energy for recreation and social obligations after the "work day" has ended. You possess the body power and Vital Force to recover rapidly from fatigue, and the stress of daily living without the aid of stimulants, drugs or alcohol. You can enjoy recharging sleep at night and awaken fit and alert.

Keeping the body totally healthy and fit is not a job for the uninformed or careless person. It requires an understanding of the body and of a healthy lifestyle and then following that lifestyle for a long, happy life! The purpose of "The Bragg Healthy Lifestyle" is to wake up the possibilities, a rebirth within you, a rejuvenation of your body, mind and spirit for a total balanced body health. It's within your reach, so start today! Daily our hearts and prayers go out to touch your heart and soul with nourishing, caring love for your total health!

With love, your health friends,

Patricia and Paul C. Bragg

Spiritual Health Promotes Physical Health

The First Step to Powerful Nerve Force: Meditation, Prayer, Faith, Forgiveness & Fears

"Be still and know that I am God." It is in the peaceful silence of meditation and prayer that you find a higher power than yourself. This power can help, guide and direct you towards the healthy goals in life you are seeking.

It is important you set aside a period twice daily – morning and evening – during this time, the mind can go into meditation and prayer to build inner strength. There must be order and clear purpose to your thinking. Silently restate your new goals in life. Remember you must displace all old, useless and damaging habits of thought with bright, new healthy ideas. Smile!

Every constructive thought stimulates the nervous system with great vitality and vigor, and this sustained and powerful activity stimulates the entire body. Through meditation and prayer you are now building a strong mind in a healthy, strong body! You are building powerful Nerve Force because you are opening that inexhaustible reservoir of energy and creative intelligence which lies within each human.

Meditation and prayer will help establish equilibrium in your mind, body and soul. It infuses you with new energy and expanded awareness, while it instills you with an inner calm and peace! You gain strength to do and to endure – to take the strains and pressures of life in stride. You will be better able to face whatever problems that may arise with sufficient Nerve Force to solve them.

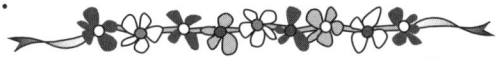

I release all the negativity within me, and open myself up to happiness and opportunity. – "50 Mantras to Start Your Day" • www.huffpost.com

Praise the Lord! He carries us in His arms daily. – Psalms 68:20

Life is a precious, beautiful song and love is the music.

Simple Techniques of Meditation & Prayer

Meditation and prayer are powerful. They allow you to analyze your life in relation to your lifestyle, environment or with a particular person, thing, field of knowledge, principle, etc. In other words, you are getting yourself set for a glorious journey toward fulfilling your goals in life. You can proceed confidently knowing you have set yourself toward a destination or goal which you will achieve with lasting, rewarding success.

Everyone has the capacity for meditation and prayer. Only minutes of daily practice are necessary to reap lasting blessings. The effects of daily meditation and prayer for what you desire and want to be can change and empower your life! Ask for it! You will notice benefits happening fast!

True meditation and prayer are completely free from mysticism and hypnotism. They offer you the ability to adjust to the fast pace of living with increased energy, self-confidence and greater peace of mind. They give glowing inner happiness and bring harmony to the mental, physical and spiritual faculties. In turn, your reservoir of Nerve Force gets fuller, healthier and stronger and your life becomes filled with daily miracles!

Your daily morning meditation and prayer gives you the chance to strengthen your resolve to completely follow The Bragg Healthy Lifestyle. Then afterwards allows you to plan your day constructively! Your evening meditation and prayer offers you the opportunity to review your day and evaluate your accomplishments and your mistakes as you plan how to correct the latter! During meditation and prayer, the body experiences a state of peaceful repose more profound than sleep. Studies have shown that the pulse, respiration and the metabolism slow down to levels below those ordinarily reached during sleep. People normally feel as refreshed following a session as they would after a nap.

I cannot overstate the importance of the habit of quiet meditation and prayer for more health of the body, mind, heart and spirit. – Patricia Bragg
"In quietness shall be your strength." – Isaiah 30:15

Meditation and Prayer Helps Master Life

Taking inventory of yourself this way is important. You will soon notice a much greater peace, tranquility and health within yourself. Life will flow more easily for you. Annoying events, things and people that used to bother you will no longer have the same effect upon you. This will give you more energy for creative thinking and living.

The release, peace and relaxation that is experienced following meditation and prayer envelopes the entire day, with a softening effect upon your entire outlook and relations with life and others. The degree of personal involvement in emotional problems is diminished. This is not to say that emotional capacity is weakened! On the contrary, this wellspring is deepened as your inner life achieves greater life balance and stability. Meditation and prayer eliminates the causes of tension in a natural way (not like toxic tranquilizers), as it subtly sharpens the mind, heart and senses. This release from mental tension and physical duress gives a healthy effect to your entire well-being. **Daily meditation and prayer helps to build a healthier balance to restore the body's normal rhythm of functions. Millions worldwide benefit from Mother Nature's wise, practical and powerful guidance and love.**

You Are What You Think and More

You will become immersed in patterns of decay if your mind is focused on negative thoughts and matters that are synonymous with disintegration. It's easy to observe the way this process works in the lives of others. It's much more difficult to see it in ourselves. Turn your mind away from negative thoughts, but not in distaste and revulsion. Rather, turn eagerly toward that which is new, fresh and desirable – remembering the wisdom gleaned from past lessons. Look ahead to the many years you will have to enjoy what and who you are, because of the experiences you are living through today. Waste no energy on recriminations or self-pity, instead move forward toward the bright future with new energy!

No man can violate Nature's Laws and escape her penalties! – Julian Johnson

Your Life is the Miracle of Miracles

You hold the miracle of miracles right now in the palm of your hand. You have the treasure of life! Think what that means to you! You are a living, breathing person! Life is the most priceless treasure on this earth. You have that treasure. Within you lies the mental power to be anything you want to be! You have a reasoning, logical mind. **Within your being you have the kingdom of heaven. Find that heaven and you have reached bliss-consciousness. You'll have found heaven on earth and life becomes so precious and wonderful!**

If you want more Nerve Force, energy and life, you will have to plan, plot and start creating, becoming and shaping your life! Look ahead. Have firm plans for living your life. Actually envision your future. You may change those plans and visions, but have them you must! Your creative force deep within you must reach out toward a bright future if you want to become one with the healthy flow of life! **Your entire mind and being will be super energized in the process to go for your goals and dreams!**

To Over-Rest is To Rust

Remember that your body will yield to your thoughts. **You are what you think!** By using your mind you sharpen its edge. Give it challenges with things to do and learn. Over-resting your mind gains nothing but its softening! Like the body, the more active you keep your mind, the better and sharper it will be. **Recent studies show:**

If you don't use it, you will lose it!

To over-rest mentally or physically is to rust. Get the negative thoughts out of your mind and demand more action from it! Let nothing and no one stop you in your quest for inner mental strength, peace and happiness!

As you follow the *Building Powerful Nerve Force* program, you will feel the flow of new power surging throughout your entire body. Summon into action your will-power and self-determination! Faithfully adhere to and work on your new positive thoughts daily. Remember, your flesh is dumb. Make your body obey your mind!

Build *"The Will to Win"* in Your Life

Life and Nerve Force flows through nerves at all times.

The more power you furnish to your nerves, the healthier and more well-balanced you will be. You'll get more out of life and have a greater chance of reaching the goals you wish to achieve! We all want to develop a strong mind in a strong body. We all want to be successful in life and reach our dreams and fulfill our life goals.

We'd like to share with you the ingredients of a winning philosophy. We've seen it proven in the successful people we have known. You've probably heard the phrase *"The Will to Win"* so many times that it has become a cliché, but stop and look at it afresh and realize its true significance. You must have this *"Will to Win"* if you are going to build powerful Nerve Force in your body. This is the indispensable first ingredient *"Will to Win"* in this healthy nerves and lifestyle program.

There's no better time to build your *"Will to Win"* than during your meditation and prayer periods. Tell yourself over and over that nothing and no one is going to stop you from building powerful Nerve Force! During your morning meditation and prayer tell yourself that you are not going to let anyone drain you of your emotional energy – no matter what they do!

If someone tries to irritate, nag or torment you, you are going to have the *"Will to Win"* over such circumstances. That *"Will to Win"* will keep you from stooping to another person's low level. Don't let anyone drag you down to their sorry level of emotional instability! It's not always possible to avoid people who are so miserable, unhappy and low in Nerve Force that they want to drag others down into the same state. Build your Nerve Force and make your *"Will to Win"* so strong that you will not be affected by these negative personalities!

Set goals and challenge yourself to meet them.

If you have been stricken by illness – your new car, your new home, your new big bank balance – all fade into unimportance until you have regained your vigor and zest for living. – Peter Steincrohn, M.D., author of: "Low Blood Sugar" and "How to Get a Good Night's Sleep"

You Need Inspiration To Guide Your Destiny

In every realm and arena of life, it is the person with a great *"Will to Win"* who makes their dreams come true. We talk about the human mind, emotions and the body. We dare say that the most important thing within each of one of us is our will. Our own actions – guided by our willpower – are what ultimately decides our destiny!

Most people live life running in circles. They waste a lot of valuable Nerve Force going nowhere fast! If you are going to be a healthy, strong and well-balanced person, you must have a well planned and healthy sense of direction. You must know where you are going. Your inner compass will guide you in the right direction and be your inspiration. Yes, you've got to have inspiration! We wish we could tell you what inspiration was – by golly then we would be the two greatest psychologists and philosophers the world has ever known!

Even people who rely most upon inspiration cannot tell you exactly what it is. Poets, artists and musicians can't tell you what inspiration is. But, we can all recognize its results! We have both seen total nervous and physical wrecks become suddenly inspired by a friend, health teacher, a book, etc. In a matter of months, they rebuilt their minds and bodies and became healthy balanced people again! They accomplished what seemed impossible!

Although we cannot define inspiration, we would like to describe one facet of what we think it means when a person is inspired. It's when people clearly see themselves – not as they are – but as they can be. It's when they see themselves – not in terms of their weaknesses, poor health, low vitality, depleted Nerve Force and failures or their inadequacies – but in terms of what they want to become!

Faith and Vision Create Miracles

When you begin to believe you can be what your inner vision tells you that you can become – that's when you're inspired. When you no longer see your weaknesses – but your strengths – then you discover the power and ability to do things you never dreamed of doing before!

During your daily meditation and prayer you must forget any inadequacies and reach inside to find your strength and true purpose – it's there! See yourself as who you want to be. Paint a vivid picture in your mind. Concentrate on that image and carry it with you daily. By following The Bragg Healthy Lifestyle, you are working with Mother Nature, powers higher than yourself! You are then living by inspiration, one of the most tremendous forces in this great universe!

Those happy, healthy, strong and vigorous people – those people who accomplish greatness – all those of faith, possess a deep spiritual philosophy. They believe that their lives are protected by a Power greater than their own. They believe there is a destiny which guides their lives. Nothing can thwart them! Following the Eternal Laws of Mother Nature they can accomplish great things!

Therapeutic Use of Forgiveness

Forgiveness sets us free from the past. Forgiveness is a process for most of us, wherein we work through grief, rage, sorrow, fear and confusion. Forgiveness comes at last as a relief and also a release for the heart. We can appreciate the truth that forgiveness is mostly for our own sake as a way to let go of any painful hurts and wrongs of the past. Forgiveness is one of the great teachings we receive in our spiritual, mental and emotional life.

HEALTHY NERVE POWER: For extra "nerve power" insurance, take daily high-stress B complex, and a multi vitamin-mineral with calcium and magnesium. Also, to relax and sleep better, try melatonin, magnesium, calcium & lemon balm (see page 70), Sleepytime herbal teas are natural relaxers that you can take before bedtime instead of sleeping pills.

Exercise is the best natural anti-anxiety agent available. It reduces tension as it relieves aggression and frustration, aids concentration and mental focus while curbing the appetite and improving sleep.

Count your blessings one by one and you will see what the Lord has done!

I give thanks for all Miracle Blessings I receive daily. – Patricia Bragg

Let Mother Nature and God Inspire You!

We'd like to urge you to ask Mother Nature to inspire you in your prayer and meditations and, while following our *Building Powerful Nerve Force Program*, to inspire you in your work, business and home. In Mother Nature you will find a power that will help you reach the heights of more healthy balanced living. Here are more great ingredients for a winning philosophy:

First: During meditations, dream great dreams and through meditation work to develop a will that translates those dreams into reality. **Develop the *"Will to Win."***

Second: Find inspiration in some great goal, some worthy cause or real challenge and let someone or something inspire you to see yourself not for what you are, but for what you can become and accomplish in life.

Third: Live by this Bragg Nerve Building Program, no matter what! Do the greatest good possible within you! Live up to the highest potential that you have! Accomplish those goals which have been set for you by Mother Nature! We know that if you meditate and pray twice to three times daily along these lines and build upon your inner strengths you will win and conquer and triumph with a long, happy, fruitful life!

The stress in our life can have mental, spiritual and physical effects upon us. One physical effect of stress is to negatively affect cholesterol synthesis, thus it can contribute to increased blockages in blood vessels. **One way to handle stress is meditation and prayer therapy. This therapeutic use can take many forms and here are steps called "Prayer, Meditation and Forgiveness."**

3 Steps – Prayer, Meditation & Forgiveness:

1. Forgiveness from others. In your meditation and prayer time say to those who come to your mind you have upset, etc., "I ask for your forgiveness."
2. Forgiveness for those who have hurt or harmed you. In meditation and prayer, offer them your forgiveness.
3. Extend a full heartfelt, loving forgiveness to yourself.

There Are Six Basic Fears

• Sickness • Poverty • Old Age
• Criticism • Loss of Love • Death

The majority of people – if asked what they fear the most – would reply, "I fear nothing." Their reply would be inaccurate, because every human being is, at some time, the victim of one or more of the six basic fears. Millions of people are crippled their entire lives by several or all of these fears. They live with high nervous tension while their Nerve Force is barely operating at a low ebb. Eventually, this causes a nervous breakdown.

Fear can attack the physical, mental, spiritual and material areas of life. It can strip you of your material possessions. In fact, fear makes difficult the tasks of procuring the bare necessities of life – food, shelter and clothing. Fear can destroy initiative, enthusiasm and ambition. It destroys your self-confidence and stifles the imagination. Fear can make you grouchy, dishonest, mean and irritable in your relationships with others!

Fear is dangerous because it generally exists in the subconscious and is not easily detected by its victim. If fear disclosed its presence by acute pain in the form of a headache, it would be less fatal. It would then be detected and its victims could eliminate it. Instead it comes like a thief in the night and poisons the mind so that it cannot function constructively for a healthy life.

You and only you can ferret out your fears and send them packing! No alibi will save you if you fail or refuse to rid yourself of fear because only one thing is required – the one thing that you control – your state of mind.

A strong state of mind is something that people acquire when they have built up large reserves of Nerve Force. Fearful thoughts are banished when there is powerful Nerve Force. This vital kind of Nerve Force cannot be purchased from any store – it must be created!

People with winning attitudes win!

With faith nothing is impossible. – Matthew 17:20

The greatest factor in pulling this country out of the doldrums of the great 1930's depression was the positive change in the minds of the American people in response to President Roosevelt's confident assurance,

"We have nothing to fear but fear itself."

A statement of timeless truth! Fear tends to paralyze. But if we face our fears intelligently, we can handle them.

Take a Hard Look at The Six Basic Fears:

Fear of Sickness

The seed of ill health lives in every human mind. To prevent this seed from blossoming into a terrible living fear, it is your duty to yourself to build your Nerve Force to its highest possible level. When the Nerve Force is very low, every ache and pain is magnified into a possible disease. The imagination runs wild. A person will have a headache and right away will imagine it's a brain tumor!

When you live The Bragg Healthy Lifestyle as outlined in this book, you'll diminish the fear of ill health. Start living The Bragg Healthy Lifestyle and as Nerve Force builds, fears will vanish!

Fear of Poverty

There can be no compromise between poverty and riches! The roads to these two extremes travel in opposite directions. If you want riches, you must refuse to accept any circumstance that leads toward poverty. The word "riches" is used here in its broadest sense and refers not only to financial wealth, but also to health, perpetual youthfulness, vitality, energy and long life – which are our physical, spiritual, mental and material estates. To us, the greatest true wealth is vigorous, vibrant health!

Fear of poverty is a state of mind brought on by Nerve Exhaustion. Build Powerful Nerve Force and you will eliminate the fear of poverty. In fact, in the process of building Powerful Nerve Force, you will already be traveling the Road to Health, which is your true wealth!

It was Confucius who said: "Eat not for the pleasure thou mayest find therein; eat to increase thy strength, eat to preserve the life thou has received from Heaven."

Fear of Old Age

When the Nerve Force drops to a low level, this great fear takes hold of the mind. It sends a cold shudder through the body of the worrier. They see themselves as old and feeble and a burden to everyone around them. They fear losing their eyesight, hearing, memory, hair and teeth and becoming weak, unattractive and senile.

This unreasonable fear of old age is one we all must fight by living The Bragg Healthy Lifestyle combined with constructive and positive thinking. Let us reason this "dilemma" out together logically and intelligently. First, there is no such thing as old age. There is not a cell in our bodies that is over 11 months old, except our bones and teeth. Every day we tear down millions of body cells and every day we build millions of new cells. So what part of us is old? The answer is – "No part of us is old!" The toxic poisons that get into our bodies, prematurely ageing us, are our main enemies – not our birthdays!

We hear this statement many times: "Man is as old as his arteries." That is definitely correct! There are many people 70, 80 and even 90 years old who have healthy flexible, clean and rust-free arteries. They have good circulation, keen eyesight and good hearing. They have learned how to keep their arteries free from clogging waste and toxic material. On the other hand, you find people in their 40s, 50s and 60s who have clogged arteries and suffer from premature ageing and health problems. **Remember there are two kinds of ages – calendar years and biological years. The calendar years mean nothing if you live by the Laws of Mother Nature! We have friends who are over 100 years old by the calendar, but are leading a life that's superior to many people in their 40s and 50s. These people have found the *Fountain of Youth* by living The Bragg Healthy Lifestyle!**

The true vocation of man is to find his way to himself.
– Hermann Karl Hesse, Swiss Poet, Nobel Prize 1946

Most everyone turns to God when in anguish, emergencies and in need.

Optimism is the faith that leads to achievements, nothing can be done without hope.
– Helen Keller, famous author who was blind, mute and deaf.

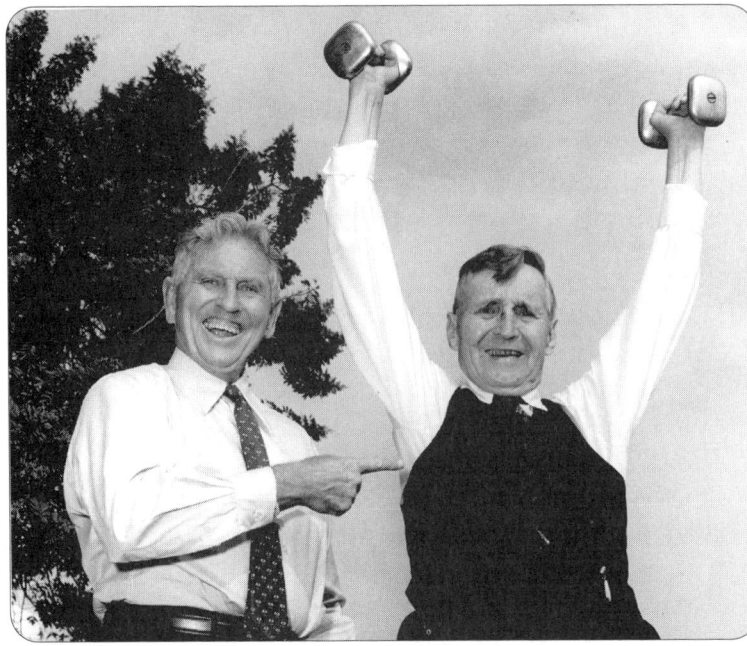

Paul C. Bragg with his youthful friend – their 'love of life' defies time!

My father's good friend, Roy White of Long Beach, CA, in his 106th year of life, had a tireless, painless and ageless body. He knew the Laws of Mother Nature and he lived by them. He didn't fear old age and was a young man in biological years. We both could name many, many more friends like Roy who in their 80s, 90s and even over 100, were biologically youthful!

Fear of Criticism

When the Nerve Force dips to a low level, one becomes extremely sensitive. Such a person feels that all eyes are upon them, ready to tear them apart with criticism. To eliminate this fear the first thing you must get into your mind is that many people are full of envy. The only way they can justify their own weakness is to constantly criticize others. Actually, such criticism is a back-handed compliment. It means that you are accomplishing something which the other person is not able to do.

A friend of ours who is a veteran of the political arena has often remarked, "If someone isn't shooting barbs at you, you aren't getting anywhere. The only time to worry is when you don't get any criticism – it means you're standing still." **Always remember that no matter what or how well you do in this life you cannot please everyone – sometimes not even your closest blood relatives!**

Dad remembers well those many years ago when some of his family and friends used to criticize him by calling him a "health nut," "food faddist," "health crank" and other more uncomplimentary names after he began to live in a healthy way. But Dad's Nerve Force was at a high level and they could not disturb his peace of mind! My father's healthy lifestyle continued to build powerful Nerve Force, resulting in vigorous health and living in a state of agelessness. He had long since buried most of his critics!

Living by wisdom and intelligence, we let criticism pass over us like water off a duck's back. We live by the finer force of Mother Nature. We are one with God and Mother Nature. Therefore, why should we let weak, uninformed minds influence us? We are living at a high rate of mental, physical and spiritual vibration. When you live by truth and intelligence, petty criticism cannot touch you! You are impervious to slander and the talk of small minds.

Fear of the Loss of Love

When your Nerve Force is at a low ebb, you are inclined to develop an inferiority complex and can easily lose your self-confidence. As you start to feel inferior you begin to fear that someone else may take away anyone who is near and dear to you. There is just one way to defeat this gnawing fear. You must build your Nerve Force so high by living The Bragg Healthy Lifestyle that any feeling of inferiority will leave you forever!

Jealousy is something all humans must fight. We can love someone, but that does not mean that we own that person. As you build your Nerve Force, you will see the wisdom of letting every person have their own personal ways. Build your Nerve Force so high that you will be above jealousy and the fear of losing your loved ones.

Love is the strongest force in the world! Give and be kind, understanding and loving, and you will be appreciated and loved more by family and friends. Remember that you can never lose one whom you loved and be thankful for the time you enjoyed and shared. With separations, hold no bitterness, as it can bring you unhappiness! You must remember that there are plenty of fickle people in the world and there is no use crying over their loss. In such cases, one might do well to remember this wise classic saying:

> ***'Tis better to have loved and lost than never to have loved at all.***

The fear of being alone and unloved – although it haunts many people – is a groundless one. There is always someone who needs your love and who needs to love you. "Seek and ye shall find." All you need is the confidence that comes with health and a powerful Nerve Force!

Fear of Death

> ***Many die many times before their death. It seems most strange that one should fear death, seeing that death, a natural transition we all face, opens up to another realm for eternity – everlasting life will come when it will come.***

Accept death as a transition years away and then pass that thought out of your mind! Let youth and your years be a preparation for a wholesome, happy future and a fulfilled life! Then there is no reason why you should not die fulfilled after a long lifetime record! If you have worked well, done your share of good and service in the world, and have your affairs in order (your *will, trust, thank-you letters maybe with voice tapes*), then when heaven calls you will be prepared with a grateful heart!

We must all face and accept death when the time arrives. All life is a preparation for that grand climax for eternity. Govern yourself and your affairs so that you can leave satisfied and hopefully, with few regrets!

Bear in mind that science has shown that the entire universe is made of mainly one thing – energy. It can be transformed, but it cannot be destroyed. Life is energy. If energy cannot be destroyed, life cannot be destroyed! Like other forms of energy, life may move through a variety of processes causing transition or change, but it remains as life energy. Death is merely a transformation. If death is not a simple change or transition, then nothing follows death except for an eternal and peaceful rest and sleep and is nothing to be feared!

Death is the furthest thing from our minds. We think in terms of living! Think like the Eskimo, who believes that as we fall asleep each night we die, only to begin an entirely fresh, new life when we wake each morning. We strive to make our days as perfect as possible!

The River of Thoughts – Positive or Negative

Life resembles a great river which splits into two different directions. One stream carries all who embark on it to inevitable success, health and happiness. The other fork of the river flows in the opposite direction, just as surely carrying those riding upon it to ill health, premature ageing, unhappiness and failure. **This river is neither fantastic nor artificial. It exists absolutely as the Mississippi does, but in the minds of humans; it flows not with water, but with thought. The success fork of the river represents positive thought; the failure stream, negative thought.** The most dangerous negative is fear!

Faith Versus Fear

Faith creates strong values! Fear destroys them. Faith builds! Fear tears down. It has been so since the dawn of civilization and it will be so until the end of time. All success has its beginning in faith. All failure has its beginning in fear. That is why we need to understand the nature and causes of fears and how to overcome them!

Remember fear need not be permanent! We say this with confidence because we've learned first-hand about the uplifting power of faith versus the destructiveness of fear. The major portion of our lives has been spent helping people in all walks of life to master fear and develop faith. Innumerable times we have had people come into our offices or one of our Health Crusades so whipped by fear that they were ready to end it all by suicide! We have also seen these same people, after following our Nerve Building Program detailed in this book, change their lives with miracles and become ready, willing and eager to attack whatever problems life placed in their paths.

"You've got to accentuate the positive, eliminate the negative, latch on to the affirmative . . ." Bing Crosby

You cannot be free of nerve tensions, stresses and strains if you are full of fear. You cannot enjoy super health and youthfulness unless you have faith in Mother Nature and yourself! You must have such complete faith in them and yourself that you can banish all of your mental and physical ills. When you build your reservoirs of Nerve Force through constructive healthy living, you can accomplish this goal of minimizing fear from your life!

Overcoming Fears

After building your Nerve Force to the highest possible level you will be able to meet and defeat many of the fears that may come into your consciousness. We fully realize that it takes physical, mental, emotional and spiritual energy to overcome fear. Although you must face, confront and overcome your own fears, you are not alone in your battle!

New studies show millions of Americans use prayer daily that blesses their lives, and hospitals find prayer works miracles.

Inspiring Words Bring Miracles

Along with The Bragg Healthy Lifestyle, you must look to a Higher Power for help to free yourself from fears, stresses, frustrations, strains and tensions. It's true – Man cannot live by bread alone! In your daily prayers you can meet with this supreme power and ask for guidance and then plan, plot and follow through for success in your life!

Don't flee from fear! Analyze it and see it as no more than a feeling. Don't be bluffed by feelings! There is an Eastern fable about a man who was being pursued by horrible dark shapes that he believed were demons. In a panic, he ran, desperately trying to escape his pursuers. At last, exhausted, he collapsed against the trunk of a tree and with wild eyes turned to face his imagined tormentors. "Destroy me!" he cried. "I can run no more!" To his amazement, the horrible shapes disappeared and evaporated like mist. They weren't demons at all, only fears of his own imagination that disintegrated when he turned the light of his eyes upon them and realized the truth!

I know the sunny side of life. My Nerve Force gives me the power to radiate sunshine in the gloomiest of times. – Paul C. Bragg, N.D., Ph.D.

Sound, Peaceful, Recharging Sleep

Second Step Towards Powerful Nerve Force

Sleep is one of the great Nerve Force builders. If you are going to have a glorious day, you must first have a splendid night of relaxed deep sleep. If you go to bed with a naturally relaxed and pleasantly tired body, a tranquil mind and a fairly empty stomach, you ought to sleep like a healthy baby! If you rise early, exercise and then give yourself healthy nourishment with natural foods, then you will surely be rewarded at night with sound and recharging sleep.

The person who is still tired and low in Nerve Force after 8 to 10 hours of sleep has usually not relaxed enough. Tense during the day, they remain unable to relax even in their sleep. Quality – not quantity – is what counts in sleep! Demand only the best and if you don't get it, ask yourself, "Why didn't I get enough sleep?"

Relaxed – Deep Sleep Must be Earned

It is impossible to get sound, relaxed sleep if you are constantly stimulating your nervous system with tobacco, coffee, tea, alcohol, sugar and cola drinks. A healthy diet of natural foods and correcting imbalances of body, mind and spirit are essential, as is open air exercise. Healthy children are physically active and the ones who play the hardest always sleep the soundest and get better grades. How can adults, who must cope with stresses, strains and tensions of modern life, expect sound, relaxed sleep when they don't get the required oxygen? If you want an excellent night's sleep, you have to earn it! You can't sit around all day eating, watching TV or working at a desk job with no exercise or outdoor activity and expect to get high quality sleep at night!

Sleep is an investment in the energy you need to be effective tomorrow." – Tom Roth

Your Mattress is Your Best Sleeping Friend

You should sleep on a firm mattress or place a board under a soft one. This allows the muscles to stretch in natural relaxation and relieves pressure on vital organs.

CHECK YOUR MATTRESS

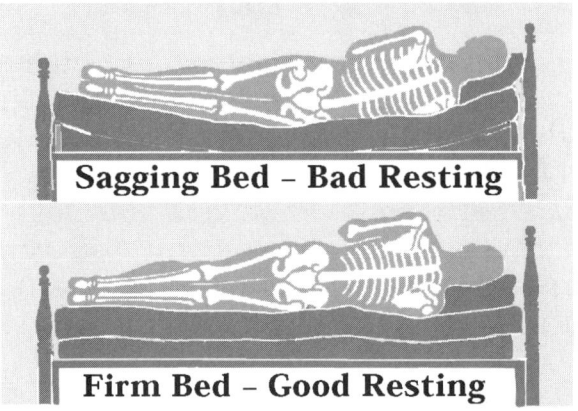

During our world health tours, we often had to move our mattresses onto the floor to be firmer. It seems that some of the world's top hotels put their money into showy lobbies and not into good firm mattresses. We also often would find old, sagging mattresses in many of the homes we visited – but new cars in their garages! At our California desert home we had new wood platforms made. A firm mattress goes on top of this board with four legs on strong casters. Try a "miracle foam" mattress pad on top of the mattress – it's great. It might take you a few nights to become accustomed to being stretched out flat, but soon your body will thank you with more energy.

We traveled all over the world in trains, planes, ships, buses, automobiles and often used soft foam ear plugs that shut out unavoidable sounds and noises. We felt it absolutely necessary that we sleep in a quiet place! Even though at times we'd fall asleep when there was noise, the vibratory action of that noise could have a direct effect on the heart, circulation and nervous system.

Nervous Tension can ruin your health in many ways and diminish your productivity and shorten your lifespan.
– Dr. Edmund Jacobson, author "You Must Relax"

Dreams Can Reflect Past and Present Life

By exerting your willpower you can eat correctly, get enough exercise and breathe deeply – but you cannot sleep soundly by willpower alone. Through activity of the body and the brain you can cause weariness – but that will not insure you perfect rest. You may be too tired or too mentally excited to sleep. If you, for example, were watching a TV movie of violence, slaying characters and solving crimes you may find sleep reluctant. Don't waste time watching TV violence – it can cause restless sleep and even bad nightmares! But, when the brain and the body are moderately and wisely used, then sweet sleep follows.

However, too much sleep is often worse than too little! You can drug yourself with sleep to the point of stupidity, causing the blood circulation in the brain to become overactive and invoke frightening dreams. Fantasy can rise from the subconscious. Dreams can plunge you into the past and may even be at times distressful. Then with weary relief we wake to reality. Yet, isn't it strange? We have our life's experiences to draw on and our dreams can vary, reflecting our experiences. **It's healthy lifestyle living with sound sleep that lets us enjoy more life-changing, uplifting, peaceful, guiding dreams.** ***www.sleeps.com***

SLEEP SHOULD NOT BE UNDERESTIMATED –

I cannot stress this enough! It's when our brains detoxify, our nervous systems, rest and our bodies heal. Without regular deep sleep, we are on track to get hormonal imbalances, weight gain, mood swings, brain fog, and so many other frustrating but preventable symptoms. Not sleeping enough is a big problem in this country: over the last 40 years Americans on average, sleep two hours less. But it's not just about quantity. Our *quality* of sleep is also suffering.
– Dr. Mark Hyman

"The nicest thing for me is sleep, then at least I can dream." – Marilyn Monroe

Read: "Dreams – Your Magic Mirror" by Elsie Sechrist

The average person spends about 23 years sleeping of a 75 year average lifespan.

Books Can Be Your Teachers & Relaxers

Govern yourself so that your sleep will be relaxed and sound. Your day should be active, including exercise, yet never fatiguing. Your dinner should be early and not too heavy. Your mind should be reposed by a few hours of reading, studying or cheerful talk before bedtime.

Be wary of TV shows, movies, and videos that are promoting crime, violence and immoral unhealthy living, etc. Watching a war, western or crime story on TV puts your nerves so on edge you could have a bad night of rolling and tossing! A travel, music or classic program is fine for the evening's pleasure. Don't watch any violence – it's poison to the brain and hinders sound relaxing sleep!

A long, quiet evening at home is the best prelude to sound, relaxed sleep! Have a shelf laden with books close to your bed. Choose books consecrated to this task like the Bible, *In His Steps* by Charles Sheldon, *In Tune with the Infinite* by Ralph Waldo Trine, *Men Who Have Walked with God* by Sheldon Cheney. Also, *Letters of Robert Louis Stevenson, The Essays of Michel de Montaigne, The Diary of Samuel Pepys* – these are always reliable. *Walden* by Henry David Thoreau, *Don Quixote* by Miguel de Cervantes and *The Diary of a Nobody* by George and Weedon Grossmith are all old friends, available night and day. Enjoy *The Prayer of Jabez* by Bruce Wilkinson, *The Mastery of Love* or *The Four Agreements* by Don Miguel Ruiz and, also the *Chicken Soup for the Soul* series – they are soul inspiring. **This list could go on for pages according to your taste. Go to your local library and choose books that feed your mind, body and spirit with strength and inspiration!**

This is why we've written Bragg Books, to guide and inspire you.

The simple act of just opening one of these subtly hypnotic volumes and turning over the pages is often enough to encourage golden slumber. Soon you feel it prudent to turn off the light. The window is open and pillow nicely adjusted. You take 10 long, deep breaths in and out slowly and give a sigh of thankfulness, and then give a prayer, letting your thoughts rise towards the heavens.

Outwitting Insomnia

If sleep be coy, you might try some simple device to woo it. A rational way is to invite sleep by imitating its rhythm. Put yourself in a position of slumber, relax absolutely and – with closed eyes – breathe in the steady rhythm of sound sleep. Shut the door of your mind as well as your eyes. If this fails, try counting up to a thousand at pulse-beat time, checking off the hundreds on your fingers. It's usually a safe bet that you will never reach the last fingers. Or lie flat on your back with arms relaxed along the sides. There is something calming about this relaxed position that produces deep sleep.

Natural Ways to Cure Insomnia

Having insomnia can leave you tired, irritable and moody; but this disruptive symptom can be cured naturally. Just follow these simple steps:

1. **Exercise!** Too little exercise can lead to insomnia. Try walking for 20-30 minutes in the morning and do yoga, Qi gong or body stretches for 20 minutes in the evening.
2. **Avoid animal proteins, sugars, refined processed foods,** cola and soft drinks for these can cause sleep problems.
3. **Eliminate all caffeine from your diet** and avoid using medicines that contain caffeine, such as Excedrin; stop caffeine for 30 days and see if your sleep improves. Take calcium and magnesium one hour before bedtime.
4. **An hour before bed soak in hot bath**, add 1 cup vinegar.
5. **Here's a natural recipe for a good night's sleep:** Soak 20 almonds, 1 Tbsp poppy seeds and 1 Tbsp pumpkin seeds in 2 cups purified water for 8 hours. (All 3 are rich in tryptophan, which increases brain's serotonin levels, helping to induce sleep.) After soaking, blend seeds in water, with 1 tsp raw honey, 100% maple syrup or blackstrap molasses until smooth. An hour before sleep, warm 1 cup blended mixture over low heat and drink.

Never hurry, never worry, live with leisure, grace and care. For it's plain that constant rushing, never gets you anywhere. – R. McCann

---

Nature never deceives us; it is we who deceive ourselves.
– Jean-Jacques Rousseau

6. **Two hours before bed have a cup of hot Valerian Herb Tea**, add raw honey or herb stevia. Or hour before bed take 1/2 - 1 tsp valerian extract in juice or a 400 - 800 mgs valerian cap. Sleep experts say valerian is most effective for falling asleep faster and staying asleep longer. It calms the nervous system, relaxes muscles and acts like a sedative since the herb binds to amino acid receptors in the brain that are linked to anxiety. *www.EveryDayHealth.com* and *www.mercola.com*

Fitness Trainers Say Days Off Benefit Fitness

You don't expect fitness trainers to say a day off from exercise is good for you. However, the body does need time to rest and repair itself. Those who cut back to 3 to 4 times weekly got better results than daily exercise.

Food and Drink – Their Effects on Sleep

Drinking too much caffeine leaves most people very nervous and sleepless at night. However, other foods and eating habits can also contribute to restless slumber.

If you're having trouble sleeping, check this list:

1. **Don't over-eat before bedtime.** A large meal one or two hours before bed tends to keep you awake, and also puts on more weight. The body is then busy digesting food and isn't ready to shut down for the night.
2. **Avoid eating heavy, high-fiber, gas producing foods late at night.** Sometimes beans, nuts, raw onions and cabbage can cause some bloating and make sound sleep difficult. Eat them earlier to allow more digestion time. *Beano* helps.
3. **Don't go to bed hungry.** A light fruit snack (*apple, banana, grapes, pear*) will keep your brain from signaling hunger to the body at night that might wake you up.
4. **No alcohol.** It interferes with the deepest, most restful sleep states, and it also dehydrates the body.
5. **Beware of all caffeine** (some green teas have caffeine). It's wise to read labels before eating and drinking so you know what you are eating! (See pages 42,94)

A good laugh and a long sleep are the best cures in the doctor's book.
– Irish Proverb

Simple Ways to Keep Stress Levels Low

- Keep a journal. Recording your feelings every day is an excellent way of getting them out of your system.
- Do some soul searching. Explore your unexamined self, through group therapy or a 12-step program.
- Meditate, pray or listen to soft music 4 to 6 times a day. These "healing times" will allow you to slow down.
- Live one hour at a time, paying close attention to your feelings. Allow them to surface, write them down, then take charge and resolve to release the wrong ones.
- Learn to love and protect your physical body. Don't waste time on negative energy! Examine negative thought messages you've been telling yourself all these years. Now change them by addressing your body with love.

Remember, your life is a series of moments where you are the Captain, you are in charge! Make the most of them all!

67% American Adults Are Sleep Deprived

A National Sleep Foundation poll taken recently discovered that sadly 67% of American adults have sleeping problems. Shockingly they found over one-third (37%) are so sleepy during the daytime that their daily activities become difficult and often interfered with. See: *SleepDisorders.about.com* and *SleepFoundation.org.*

Over the past 100 years, we've reduced our average sleep time by 20% and, over the last 25 years, added an additional month to our annual work/commute time. Thus, our national "sleep debt" is rising and while our society has changed, our physical bodies and needs have not. We are paying a dear price for such "progress!"

Are You Getting Enough Sleep Lately?

The odds are you aren't getting sufficient sleep. American adults presently average 7 hours nightly. While everyone's sleep needs vary, most scientific research and studies indicate that we require 8 hours of sleep nightly.

Few are lucky enough to enjoy 5 to 6 hours of sleep and still perform well at work. To just get "caught-up," a full ten hours of rest is frequently needed and called for!

Try Lemon Balm Tea for a Night So Calm

First, make a clear and conscious choice about how you wish to spend the sixty minutes that precede your actual going to bed time. Avoid a rush to "get things ready for tomorrow" or to catch up on tasks not completed during the day. This is a time to relax and rest your body and mind. Try an aroma herbal bath or a self massage while showering, one hour before bed – it's so relaxing. Enjoy a warm soothing apple cider vinegar drink with cinnamon and honey (recipe on page 108) or soothing Lemon Balm herbal tea 1-2 hours before bedtime.

Lemon Balm, whose scientific name is *Melissa officinalis*, is a cooling plant with both nervine and antiseptic relaxing qualities. It's a member of the Labiatae family, which also includes peppermint and spearmint, lemon balm is native to most areas of Europe and is now widely grown worldwide. Flowering between June and October, it's lemon-like fragrance is unmistakable and makes a delicious tea.

Like restful chamomile, lemon balm's primary, volatile oil makes the plant medicinal. While appearing to be just a simple plant, it delivers a wide range of potent aids for complaints ranging from stomach pain to the worst cases of insomnia. Try lemon balm tea after meals and before bed, miraculous results have been reported. Also, try blending with a variety of herbal teas. Some others to try for sound sleep are: *Sleepytime*, Skullcap, and Valerian Herbal Teas, available at health stores. Also try magnesium and calcium supplements and melatonin (1-3 mg) or its tea 1-2 hours before bed. Record results in *Daily Journal* (see page 104).

Good Sleep is the Cornerstone of Health

Eight hours per night is the optimal amount of sleep for most adults. Science has established that a deficit of sleep can have serious, far reaching effects on your health!

An effective herbal sleep remedy is Chamomile Tea. Lavender and Hibiscus teas are good sleep inductors. Be cautious of drinking tea which contains stimulants or caffeine.

Interrupted or Impaired Sleep Can:

- Dramatically weaken your immune system
- Accelerate tumor growth with severe sleep dysfunctions
- Cause a pre-diabetic state, making you feel hungry and overeat that can wreak havoc on your weight
- Seriously impair your memory. Even a single night of poor sleep (4-6 hours) can impact your ability to think clearly
- Impair your performance on physical or mental tasks
- Can also increase stress-related disorders including: heart disease, stomach ulcers, constipation, and mood disorders, personality upsets and depression

Healthful Tips for Sound, Recharging Sleep

Excerpts from Dr. Mercola – www.mercola.com

The good news is there are many natural techniques you can learn to restore your "sleep health." Whether you have difficulty falling asleep or feel inadequately rested when waking up, you can find relief from these tips below:

• **Sleep in complete darkness.** Even the tiniest bit of light in the room can disrupt your internal clock and your pineal gland's production of melatonin and serotonin. Little bits of light pass directly through your optic nerve to your hypothalamus, which controls your biological clock. Light signals your brain that it's time to wake up and start preparing your body for ACTION!!!

• **Wear an eye mask to block out light.** It is not always easy to block out every stream of light using curtains or blinds.

• **Keep your bedroom temperature lower (60-65°F is best for sleeping!)** Scientists state a cooler bedroom is more conducive to sleep since it mimics the body's natural temperature drop.

• **Check bedroom for Electro-Magnetic Fields (EMFs).** EMF's can disrupt the pineal gland and production of melatonin and serotonin. Before bed unplug any phones or electronics near the bed, even when staying in hotels!

• **Turn off cell phones, move alarm clocks and other electric devices away from bed.** Light and EMF's can disturb sleep. Historically, people went to bed shortly after sundown, as most animals do, which is what nature intended for humans as well.

• **Get to bed as early as possible.** Your body recharges between the hours of 11 pm and 1 am. Also, your gallbladder dumps toxins during this same period. If you are awake, the toxins back up into your liver, which can further disrupt your sleep and your health.

• **Establish a good bedtime routine.** This could be meditation, deep breathing, aromatherapy, essential oils or a massage.

• **Don't drink fluids two hours before bedtime.** This helps reduce the likelihood or lessens frequency of needing to use the bathroom at night. Also try to empty your bladder or use the toilet right before you go to bed.

• **Have a high-protein drink/shake several hours before bed.** This helps provide L-tryptophan needed for your melatonin and serotonin production (SlimFast, Ensure).

• **Avoid before-bed snacks, particularly grains and sugars.**

• **Take a hot bath, shower or sauna before bed.** The temperature drop from getting out of the bath or shower helps to signal your body it's time for bed and sleep.

• **Wear socks to bed.** Study shows wearing socks reduces night wakings. You could put hot water in a glass bottle near your feet at night. It's so comforting!

• **Put work away at least one hour before bed.** This gives your mind a chance to unwind so you can go to sleep feeling calm, not hyped up or anxious about tomorrow's deadlines.

• **No TV one hour before bed.** TV disrupts your pineal gland function.

• **Keep a Daily Journal.** (See page 104). Write in the morning when your brain is functioning at its peak and cortisol levels are high.

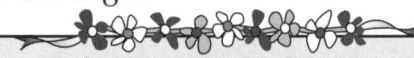

For Relaxing Delights Try These:

SIGHT: *Soften lights, close eyes and visualize beautiful nature scenes.*

SOUND: *Soothing music increases the healing and helps reduce the stress hormone cortisol by 25%.*

SMELL: *Aroma bath or shower, use a few drops of essential oils over skin. Try lemon, chamomile, lavender or sandalwood. These all have calming, relaxing effects.*

TOUCH: *Get a massage or give yourself one in the bath or shower. Lightly dab olive or coconut oil over your body, then massage feet, neck, shoulders, arms and legs for relaxing health therapy.*

Lifestyle Suggestions That Enhance Sleep

- Avoid stimulants: caffeine (in coffee, some teas, even green teas, soft drinks, chocolate, sugar) and nicotine (found in cigarettes and other tobacco products).
- Don't drink alcohol to "help" you sleep, it's unhealthy!
- Have herbal teas – anise, lemon balm, Sleepytime, chamomile (beware some Green Teas have caffeine), or try melatonin, tryptophan (5HTP), valerian, calcium and magnesium supplements; they work miracles.
- Exercise regularly, but try to be finished with your workout no sooner than 2 hours prior to bedtime.
- Avoid foods you may be sensitive to. Reactions can cause excess congestion, gastrointestinal upset, bloating or gas.
- Associate your bed with needed recharging sleep – it's wise not to sit on it to work or watch TV. *Try a memory 2" foam topper (so comfortable) on your firm mattress.*
- If you suffer from insomnia, don't nap during the day. Remember, earn better sleep by exercise and day activity.

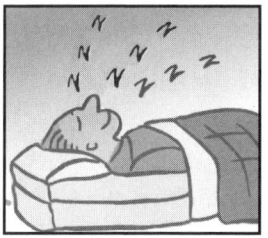

Relief for Snorer in the House

Now there are choices in treatment for relieving stubborn snoring. A simple doctor laser treatment or *Somnoplasty*, a minimally invasive procedure that can be performed as an in-office surgery. But first try nasal strips (adhesive band-aid-like device) that helps keep open nose's nasal passages and allows easier airflow during sleep. Available at pharmacies, sizes small to large. The second is RIPSNORE™, a simple, one-piece device that molds to the shape of your mouth. The device is very flexible when being fitted. It stops snoring or drastically reduces snoring in 98% of people who started using it. The RIPSNORE™ holds your lower jaw slightly forward, moving your base of tongue away from the back of your airway and soft palate – allowing your throat to be opened and the snore to be silenced. The device is almost identical to dental ones, but is obviously more affordable. *www.RipSnore.com.*

The Lord gives rest and strength to those who are weary. – Isaiah 40:29

A recharging, peaceful good night sleep is vitally important!

Stanford's Suggestions for Improving Sleep

According to Derek Loewy, Ph.D., former co-director of the Stanford Sleep Disorders Clinic's Insomnia Program, the first group therapy program for insomnia in the U.S., "Our insomniacs tend to be those with the thickest medical charts." Loewy suggests that if you don't fall asleep quickly, get out of bed and do something relaxing and enjoyable. He also advocates breathing exercises that promote relaxation and help patients deal with their sleep deficit. Loewy's program shuns drugs, "Although sedatives can induce sleep, they lose effectiveness as the body develops tolerance and addiction becomes a possibility." **Here are more suggestions:**

1. **Have set times for waking up and also going to bed, it helps the body's sleep-wake cycle settle into a regular rhythm.**
2. **Stop caffeine, especially in afternoons and evenings.**
3. **Don't drink alcohol at night, it suppresses both deep sleep and dream sleep. It may allow you to fall asleep more easily, but you're likely to suffer sleep disruption several hours later. Alcohol has many ill side-effects.**

Remember sleep comes to the body when it's relaxed. When you lie down on your bed, let your body relax until you seem to sink down through the mattress and through the floor and beyond. **Let go of all muscular and mental tension – this is the secret of sound sleep!**

The art of muscular relaxation should be practiced throughout the day. To understand the reason for this practice, note the furrowed brow of most business people, the tensely clasped hands of the nervous woman or the strained look of city dwellers. Everyone who is subjected to nervous tension, stress or strain – regardless of their occupation – should have periods for muscular relaxation during the day. If someone does fine work requiring constant use of their eyes, they should relax their eye muscles by looking away at distant objects. A writer should leave the computer to tidy the office or take a rest. Whatever your work, change your set of duties several times a day. Take a few moments at regular intervals to completely relax all the muscles of your body. Go limp, close your eyes and think pleasant, cheerful thoughts.

The Luxury of the Siesta

Spain, Switzerland, Mexico, France, Italy, South America and many other countries are highly advanced when it comes to relaxation! They have a rest period in the middle of the day. They eat their lunch, then lie down for a deep, relaxing rest and sleep. Blessings and praises to the founders of this custom! This healthy custom – which years ago was prevalent throughout our own Southern States – has unfortunately become banished by modern Americans now. The abandonment of the afternoon nap is a high price to pay for so-called progress!

My father and I always enjoyed our daily siesta – the "40 winks" after lunch. When we awoke after our short after-lunch snooze, we felt that we're beginning a whole fresh new day! The midday siesta (30-60 minute snooze) gives you two days in one! It will recharge your batteries and send you back into the game of life with renewed vigor! If either one of us had ever become President of the U.S., our first official proclamation would have been, "A one and a half hour healthy midday break for all!"

Digestively speaking, your stomach requires what is known as the eupeptic pause after eating. For a short time after lunch and dinner, let your stomach have the center stage so your energy can fully concentrate on digesting the meal you just gave it. Allow the body to supply energy to your stomach as exclusively as possible.

Try Power Nap For Miracle Recharge

It's very typical for some people to experience low energy levels around mid-afternoon. Many people are sleep-deprived which also adds to low energy levels. Even a 20-30 minute nap after work will leave you far more refreshed and alert for the evening than anything else. But avoid sleeping too long because you can run the risk of not being sleepy for your normal bedtime.

HEALTHY MIND HABIT: Wake up and say – Today I am going to be happier, healthier and wiser in my daily living! I am the captain of my life and I am going to steer it to living a 100% healthy lifestyle! Fact is happy people look younger and have fewer health problems! – Patricia Bragg

How to Have Deep, Sound, Relaxed Sleep

Let your sleeping tonic be composed of exercise in fresh air and sunshine. You do not get sound, healthy sleep when you take a sleeping drug – you simply get drugged! It's a vicious habit which may lead you toward a complete nervous breakdown. These drugs are both addictive and dangerous. As time goes on, habitual drug users must resort to increased dosages. These pills can – and do – kill!

Always keep in mind that tobacco, coffee, tea and cola drinks can cause sleeplessness! A heavy meal in the late evening can also give you a poor night's rest.

You should sleep on a firm mattress. This helps to stretch muscles in natural relaxation. What wonderful sleep you get when your muscles and bones are held securely in place! Your sleeping space should be at least 36 inches in width. If you have a sleeping partner, the bed should be 72 inches wide or a queen or king size.

At the rate of eight hours of sleep per every 24-hour period, we spend a third of our lives in bed. With this in mind, get yourself the best bed and bedding you can buy. Remember that its value is not necessarily determined by the sum you pay, but by the quality of restoring sleep it gives you!

Wear comfortable cotton or silk nightclothes, if any. There is a delicious freedom and freshness in sleeping naked, especially in the summertime.

A night of sound, peaceful, relaxing, refreshing and rejuvenating sleep is your finest health insurance! Woo sleep. Work to win it. Let it fill your body's reservoirs with powerful Nerve Force. Sleep is one of your best friends! Sleep is kind, it heals and recharges your Nerve Force.

Avoid drinking too many liquids in the evening. Drinking lots of water, juice or tea may result in frequent bathroom trips throughout the night. Be careful of caffeinated drinks, which act as diuretics, that only make things worse.

Lavender helps you relax. Before drying off after your night bath or shower, place three drops of lavender essential oil on a damp washcloth and rub it gently over your body. The soothing active agents in the lavender oil will enter into your body through your skin and nose.

Natural Healthy Food

Third Step Towards Powerful Nerve Force

A happy life consists of tranquility of the mind. The instrument of the mind is the brain, which is part of the physical body. It's impossible to have this tranquility of the mind if the brain is suffering from malnutrition.

Most brains in our society today are undernourished. Never before in history have we had so many mentally challenged children! Never before have we had so many people suffering from mental disease! **A traveler from outer space would look down on the earth and say,** ***"What a mess you have made of your beautiful planet!"***

What we must do is equip ourselves to withstand the effects of the pressures we encounter. To do this, we must build powerful Nerve Force. Our Central Nervous System – with the brain as its center – must be strengthened and kept healthy with proper nourishment! One of the most critical factors closely related to the health of the Central Nervous System is the B-Complex vitamins. When the body has adequate amounts of healthy nutrients (page 122), it can then withstand the stress, strain and tension that our mile-a-minute life can often cause!

However, our modern "dead" foods are sadly lacking in these vital ingredients! Since the civilized diet has very little vital B-Complex vitamins, our bodies suffer from the same deficiency. No wonder the world is sick!

The Bragg Healthy Lifestyle Eating Habits

You need to learn not only what to leave out of your diet, but also importantly, what you should put into it. You will find that you can nourish your body without sacrificing meal-time enjoyment once you understand the basic health principles of proper nourishment. **This health knowledge shows you elements your body needs to build, develop and live healthy as it was meant to do naturally! Combinations of healthful foods packed with vital nutrients are abundant worldwide.**

The first step, of course, is to get into *the habit of eating for health.* Such a habit is not difficult to form. Although the instinctive sense of food selection has been submerged with all the advertising of the popular fast, junk foods, etc. You have to be strong minded! Like any other ability or skill, a healthy lifestyle must be kept constantly in practice or its powers will deteriorate. Only by exercising this natural health instinct and desire can we revive and strengthen our health.

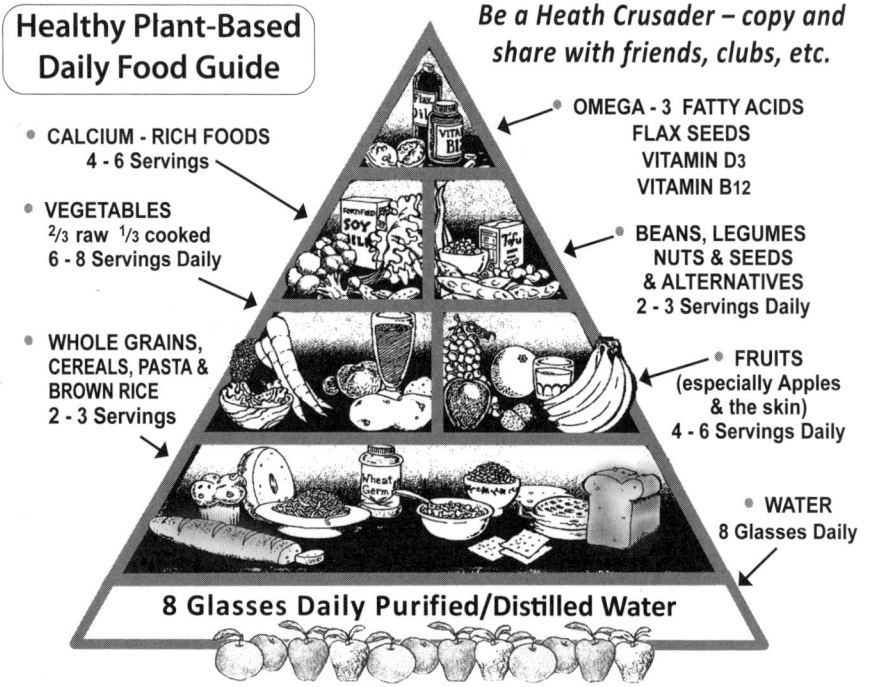

The *Healthy Plant-Based Daily Food Guide Pyramid* **illustration above represents an ideal way of eating for achieving optimal nutrition, health and longevity!** You will notice that this Food Guide Pyramid is based on healthy organic plant-based foods, with emphasis on fruits, vegetables, whole grains, vegetable protein foods, non-dairy calcium foods, raw nuts, seeds and purified water. This is the best diet for building a healthy nervous system, disease prevention and to enjoy longevity. ***Eating a diet based on these dietary guidelines will help provide the nutrients you need for optimal health!***

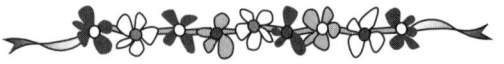

What a person eats becomes his own body chemistry.

Purified or Distilled Water: Is the pyramid's foundation. We recommend drinking *pure distilled water* as it is the best type of water for the body. Drink at least eight – 8 oz glasses of distilled water daily and even more if lifestyle sports, work, etc. requires it. Read *Water – The Shocking Truth,* see page 218.

Whole Grains: Whole grains are the next pyramid level. Avoid all GMO processed, refined grain products and eat only unrefined, whole grain bread and cereal products. Grains such as whole wheat, brown rice, oats, millet, quinoa, and 100% whole grain breads and cereals are the best. One serving of whole grains is equal to 1 slice of whole grain bread, 1 ounce ready-to-eat whole grain cereal, 1 cup cooked whole grains such as brown rice, oatmeal or other grains, 1 cup whole wheat, rice, pasta or noodles, or 1 ounce other whole grain products. We recommend eating 2-3 servings of whole grains a day.

Vegetables: We recommend eating as many of your vegetables organic and raw (uncooked, in salads, juices, smoothies, etc.) as possible! When cooking vegetables, do not overcook them. Steaming or lightly stir frying is best. The more colorful rainbow of vegetables you eat, the better they are for your health as they contain more valuable nutrients and healthy phytochemicals (page 91). Eat a wide variety of organic vegetables daily. One vegetable serving is equal to 1 cup cooked vegetables or 1 cup raw uncooked vegetables, 1 cup salad, 3/4 cup vegetable juice. We recommend having 6-8 or more vegetable servings daily.

Fruits: Like vegetables, the more colorful the fruits the better they are for you. Enjoy organic fruits as much as possible! One serving of fruit is equal to 1 medium apple, banana, orange, pear or other fruit, 1/2 cup fruit, 1/2 cup of fruit juice or 1/4 cup dried fruit. We recommend eating 4-6 servings or more of organic fruits daily.

There's no substitute for a healthy diet of organic fruits, vegetables, grains and legumes. Vitamin deficiency occurs after many weeks or months of intake below recommended levels. – Complete Guide to Natural Healing

---

Junk foods, processed meats, hot dogs, sausage, sugar and fast foods can increase inflammation in your body which could lead to chronic disease. – Dr. Bob Martin, author "Secret Nerve Cures" • www.DoctorBob.com

Calcium Foods: Are plant-derived calcium-rich foods. Plant sources of calcium are healthier than dairy products because they don't contain saturated fats or cholesterol (for more info on calcium see pages 85-89). Health calcium-rich foods are: soymilk, tofu, broccoli and green leafy vegetables. Serving sizes of plant-derived calcium-rich foods include: 1 cup soymilk, 1/2 cup tofu, 1/3 cup almonds, 1 cup cooked or 2 cups of high calcium raw greens (kale, collards, broccoli, bok choy or other Chinese greens), 1 cup of calcium-rich beans (e.g. soy, white, navy, Great Northern), 1/2 cup seaweed, 1 tablespoon blackstrap molasses, 5 or more figs. We recommend having 4-6 servings of healthy non-dairy sources of calcium rich foods daily.

Beans and Legumes: Are the healthy protein foods. Vegetable protein foods are more optimal compared to animal protein foods (vegetable protein chart – page 99). Vegetable proteins do not contain artery clogging saturated fats and cholesterol found in animal foods. They do contain protective factors to prevent heart disease, cancer and diabetes. Vegetable proteins provide the body with the essential amino acids that it requires. One serving of vegetable protein foods include: 1 cup cooked legumes (beans, lentils, dried peas), 1/2 cup firm tofu or tempeh, 1 serving of "veggie meat" alternative (veggie burger patty), 3 tablespoons nut or seed butter, 1 cup soy milk. We recommend 2-3 or more vegetable protein servings daily.

Essential Nutrients: The essential and healthy fats, like Omega-3's and vitamins and minerals. Servings of healthy fats include: 1 tsp. flaxseed oil (flaxseed is high in phytonutrients called lignans), 1 Tbsp of organic extra-virgin olive oil, and 3 Tbsps raw walnuts. Other healthy essentials include nutritional B-Complex supplements that provide extra vitamin B12. Provide your body with the nutritional supplements your body requires for optimal health and longevity (page 122).

Organic natural foods are the greatest source for staying healthy!
– Patricia Bragg, Pioneer Health Crusader

Nutrition directly affects growth, development, reproduction, and well-being of an individual's physical and mental condition. Health depends upon nutrition more than on any other single factor. – Dr. William H. Sebrell, Jr.

Bad Nutrition – #1 Cause of Sickness

"Diet-related diseases account for 68% of all deaths."
– Dr. C. Everett Koop

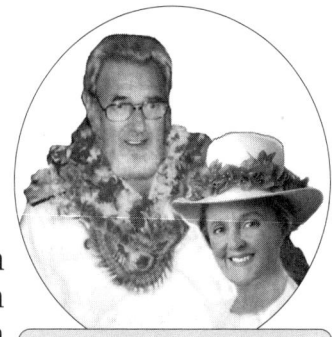

Dr. Koop & Patricia
Hawaii Health Conference

America's former Surgeon General and our friend, said this in his famous 1988 landmark report on the nutrition and health in America. People don't die of infectious conditions as such, but of malnutrition that allows germs to get a foothold in sickly bodies. Also, bad nutrition is usually the cause of non-infectious, fatal or degenerative conditions. **When the body has its full nutrition quota of vitamins and minerals, plus potassium, it's almost impossible for germs to get a foothold in a healthy, powerful bloodstream and tissues!**

You Are Exactly What You Eat and Drink

Of all the various causes of nervous exhaustion and the entire ensemble of conditions that arise with it, incorrect diet probably leads the group! If there is any one thing that must be changed before the body can respond with vigorous health and unlimited Nerve Force, it's the S.A.D. = Standard American Diet. To help relieve stress and tensions that threaten our lives, we must **eat adequate amounts of natural, healthy foods to supply the body with the important nutrients for building an active brain in a strong, healthy body.**

The Central Nervous System is made and maintained by the food you eat! How can you build a strong Nervous System and maintain it on hot dogs, washed down with caffeine-filled coffee or colas? How can greasy french fried potatoes supply the nervous system with the valuable nutrients that it needs? It cannot!

It's strange that some men will drink and eat anything put before them, but will check very carefully the oil they put in their car.

No man can violate Mother Nature's Laws and escape her penalties.

As we have devitaminized and demineralized our daily foods we have weakened our Central Nervous System. We are surrounded by an avalanche of chemicals which are poisonous and injurious to our health! Our foods are sprayed with poisonous insecticides. Then the food processors incorporate hundreds of food additives and chemicals which may make their products have longer shelf life, but will ultimately also shorten human life.

The tragic price we pay for our destruction of the B-Complex vitamins in our "civilized" foods is evident in the confusion and discouragement – combined with the nervousness and excessive fatigue – so common in our lives and world today. In our opinion the excessive use of tobacco, alcohol, coffee, tea, cola drinks and drugs is directly related to a deficiency in B-Complex vitamins! We have carefully studied the dietary habits of people who use these powerful stimulants and drugs and found in every case that these people are suffering from B-Complex vitamin deficiency.

Millions Suffer Vitamin B-Complex Deficiency

People of every age go about their daily business with their vital energies barely above the point of exhaustion. Watch carefully what they eat and you will find they are not eating foods that help to build Nerve Force.

As is typical of a deficiency, the body signals its need for nutrients with cravings. In the case of B-Complex vitamin deficiency, the body signals its craving for food. Through ignorance, however, people often seek to supply this need with incorrect material by stuffing it with the so-called "quick energy" concoctions that contain refined white sugar; such as candy, chewing gum, cakes, cookies, cola drinks, ice cream, pies and other rich, sugary desserts. These may give an apparent temporary "lift," but this false energy is quickly consumed by the body, leaving the real deficiency even greater than before. **So whenever you feel what you interpret as a "craving for sweets" – look to your nerves and reach for B-Complex vitamin supplements instead of sweets and the sugar bowl!**

A B-Complex vitamin deficiency is insidious and difficult to detect. Apparently, the troubles seem to be minor – occasional headaches, some colds and joint and stomach pains, or a clogged bowel which has to be whiplashed with a powerful drug laxative. Ask most people suffering from this deficiency, "How are you feeling today?" Since the trouble seems to be minor, their reply will usually be, *I feel great!* They have had the ailment so long that they have learned to live with it and think nothing of it.

So many people have not the slightest idea what "feeling great" really means! They go on their merry way until Mother Nature finally will not take any more abuses, and they have a complete nervous body breakdown.

Folic Acid Helps Protect the Blood

Folic acid plays a vital role in the smooth functioning of a healthy body. Long revered as a brain food, it's needed for growth of red and white blood cells and the body's energy production. Deficiencies of folic acid, B6 and B12 can lead to serious conditions such as depression, anxiety, insomnia, immune system problems and dangerously high homocysteine levels. **Two must-read books by Kilmer S. McCully, M.D. *The Homocysteine Revolution* and *The Heart Revolution* educate the reader about the deadly toxic effects of high homocysteine levels and the tragic results to the cardiovascular system.**

High Homocysteine Can Cause Alzheimer's Diabetes and Heart Health Problems

High homocysteine levels and dietary deficiencies of vitamins B6, B12, folic acid and CoQ10, can damage cells that line the blood vessel walls, setting the stage for future cardiovascular disease and increasing problems with Alzheimer's, diabetes, osteoporosis and kidney diseases. **When having a physical, demand a blood panel test that includes your homocysteine level. Dr. McCully says the safest level is 6 to 8 mcm/L, other studies agree.**

For every 10% rise in homocysteine levels, there's an equal risk of developing severe coronary disease and osteoporosis. In patients with heart disease, the risk of death 4-5 years after diagnosis, was related to the amount of homocysteine in the plasma. Everyone produces this substance naturally, but the homocysteine level can dangerously rise with heavy meat eating and when the body is sluggish (*lack of exercise, fruits, vegetables, water, etc.*), it then fails to convert it to safe, non-damaging amino acids.

In most cases, therapy with various B vitamins and a healthy menu of fresh organic fruits and vegetables offers the B vitamins necessary to reduce high homocysteine levels. But the Standard American Diet "S.A.D." doesn't supply enough B vitamins to adequately detoxify homocysteine. This has been scientifically documented by Dr. McCully.

B Vitamins & Folic Acid Are Heart Protectors

Dr. Kilmer S. McCully pioneered "The Homocysteine Revolution." Here are more positive facts from him: *"high homocysteine levels are easily corrected in most people with B-vitamins. B6, B12 and folic acid help reduce homocysteine levels. This is especially important for those who are at risk for cardiovascular problems, because 1 in every 3 people with cardiovascular disease have dangerously high homocysteine levels (safe level is 6-8 mcm/L)."* Godfrey P. Oakley, M.D., formerly with the U.S. Centers for Disease Control & Prevention, says, *"there is strong evidence from over 200 studies that increased intake of folic acid (from food or supplements) help prevent heart disease."*

In addition to supplements, folic acid is found in dates, brown rice, mushrooms, spinach, asparagus, lima beans, broccoli, oranges and cabbage. Folic acid works best taken with vitamin C, B6 and B12, and CoQ10.

Some doctors prescribe short-term relief to sufferers of angina with nitroglycerin (nitrolingual) spray and digitalis (foxglove) medications. Both increase blood flow to the heart, but in different ways. The former relaxes the veins, increasing blood supply to the heart. The latter makes the heart muscles contract more forcefully (see page 122). It's important to keep in mind that these merely offer temporary relief. The best healthy heart results come from living The Bragg Healthy Lifestyle.

Foods Rich in the B Vitamin Family

You must plan your meals to be sure that you get all of the B-family vitamins. There are so many delicious foods that will give you this all-important factor in building powerful Nerve Force. Here are some main ones:

- **Raw nuts and seeds**, provide vital B-Complex vitamins including riboflavin, niacin, thiamin, vitamin B6 and folates, essential for optimum health.
- **Whole Grains** such as barley, rye, buckwheat, spelt, teff, oatmeal, quinoa, millet, amaranth, wild rice.
- **Beans (fresh or dried), Legumes and Lentils:** such as lima beans, soy beans, green beans, as well as peas.
- **Raw Wheat Germ and Rice Bran**
- **Vegetables and Greens** such as collards, turnip, kale, spinach mustard greens, broccoli and cabbage.
- **Fruits:** oranges, grapefruits, bananas, avocados, peaches, cantaloupe. Also prune and pineapple juices.
- **Mushrooms** all varieties, fresh and dried.
- **Herbs** alfalfa, cayenne, chamomile, eyebright, fennel, ginseng, parsley, peppermint, sage, rose hips, and many more.
- **Molasses** Blackstrap.

Your Nerves Need Plenty of Calcium

We are generally more deficient in calcium than in any of the 30 other minerals the body needs to maintain health and sufficient Nerve Force. Calcium levels in the correct proportion give us sound teeth, strong bones, nerves of steel, good muscle and skin tone, a regular heart beat, an erect posture, a sharp mind and healthy vital organs. If your blood calcium level drops too much you may become nervous, cross, moody, depressed, grouchy and irritated. Calcium helps control your health and moods as it shapes your entire personality.

Calcium deficiency is a major contributing cause to the adverse changes in personality that are the result of low Nerve Force.

Calcium is all-important for proper functioning of the nerves. This mineral helps to transport impulses through the nerves from one part of the body to the other. Without calcium, you would not be able to pull your hand away from a hot stove, get out of the way of an oncoming car or even taste the food you eat! Calcium deficiency may cause cramps or convulsions, heart palpitations or a slow pulse. Calcium also helps maintain the body's delicate acid-alkaline balance.

Calcium deficiencies can be readily recognized by stunted growth, decayed teeth and brittle or porous bones which show up in X-rays. It is more difficult, however, to recognize calcium deficiencies that produce changes in the soft tissues. Yet these are the warning signs which we must learn to detect in order to prevent unnecessary misery and physical handicaps.

Only 1% of the body's calcium is used by the soft tissues. But if this essential 1% is lacking it flashes a danger signal of calcium deficiency. The most noticeable sign is extreme nervousness. Without the proper amount of calcium in the blood, the nerves cannot send messages. Tension and strain result. It is impossible for the body to relax. This is apparent in children who are highly emotional. It shows first in a mean and unpleasant disposition, fretful crying and temper tantrums which can develop into muscular twitching, spasms and even convulsions.

Calcium Deficiencies Cause Nervous Habits

Both adults and children reveal calcium deficiencies through nervous habits – such as biting the fingernails, continuous restless movements of hands and feet, constant gum chewing, picking at the nose and ears or scratching the head continually. They cannot sit still for any length of time, and there is often an uncontrollable trembling of hands and fingers – especially in adults. People deficient in calcium are usually quite irritable, flying off the handle at the slightest provocation and often going into an emotional tantrum. They may experience spells of uncontrollable weeping and be inclined to wallow in self pity. They are also "jumpy" and become upset or alarmed at the slightest noise.

Fortunately the opposite is also true. During our long experience in the field of Natural Living, we have seen the meanest, grouchiest, most irritable and nervous people undergo a personality change for the better – a transformation into happy, friendly, self-reliant people – after they change their way of living and following the wonderful and wise Health Laws of Mother Nature.

You too can make some great improvements in your life and personality by obeying the Laws of Mother Nature. Remember that you first have to live with yourself. We know you do not wish to live with an unhappy, restless and irritable person. It's your birthright to be happy and feel healthy all the time! But it is strictly an "inside job." It's #1 on the do-it-yourself list. If you are not a well adjusted and happy person, then you should start today to do something about it! Having put in over 95 combined years of research and study on this subject, we believe we can help you to help yourself to build powerful Nerve Force and a happier life.

To help you plan your meals so that you get plenty of calcium in your daily diet, here is a list of the foods that are richest in this important mineral. Do your best to get some of these foods into your diet daily.

Calcium Content Chart of Some Common Foods

Calcium Food Source	mgs	Calcium Food Source	mgs
Almonds, 1 oz.	80	Kohlrabi, (steamed) 1 cup	40
Artichokes, (steamed) 1 cup	51	Mustard Greens, 1 cup	138
Beans, (kidney, pinto, red) 1 cup	89	Oatmeal, 1 cup	120
Beans, (great northern, navy) 1 cup	128	Orange, 1 large	96
Beans, (white) 1 cup	161	Prunes, 4 whole	45
Blackstrap Molasses, 1 Tbsp	137	Raisins, 4 oz.	45
Bok Choy, (steamed) 1 cup	158	Rhubarb, (cooked) 1 cup	105
Broccoli, (raw/steamed) 1 cup	178	Rutabaga, (steamed) 1 cup	72
Brussel Sprouts, (steamed) 1 cup	56	Sesame Seeds, (unhulled) 1 oz	381
Cabbage, (raw/steamed) 1 cup	50	Soybeans, 1 cup	73
Cauliflower, (raw/steamed) 1 cup	34	Soymilk, fortified	150
Collards, (steamed) 1 cup	152	Spinach, (raw/steamed) 1 cup	244
Figs, (5 medium)	135	Tofu, firm 1/2 cup	258
Kale, (raw/steamed) 1 cup	180	Turnip greens, 1 cup	198

Sources: *Back to Eden*, Jethro Kloss; *Health Nutrient Bible*, Lynne Sonberg; website: www.vrg.org/nutrition/calcium, chart by Brenda Davis, R.D.

Benefit From Natural Foods Rich in Calcium

There are some very fine sources of calcium other than milk. Scientists feel that the most bio-available form of calcium supplement is calcium citrate. We prefer calcium found in kale, spinach, corn, beans, veggies, soy tofu and sesame seeds. In fact, as Dr. Lynch and Dr. Neal Barnard point out, all natural foods contain appreciable amounts of calcium. The chart on the previous page shows foods that contain large amounts of calcium you should include in your diet. Read these two books on milk and why it is best to avoid milk: *Mad Cows and Milk Gate* by Virgil Hulse, M.D.; and *Milk, the Deadly Poison* by Robert Cohen. Also visit these websites: *www.NotMilk.com* and *pcrm.org* (Physicians Committee for Responsible Medicine).

Milk is Not a Good Source of Calcium

Nearly everyone has the idea that the problem of calcium deficiency will be solved if they just drink milk. This is not completely true. Practically all milk in the U.S. is pasteurized, which robs and greatly reduces the availability of milk's calcium.

Dr. Harold D. Lynch – famous author, researcher and physician – said, ***"almost fanatic use of milk as a beverage has added more complications than benefits to child nutrition. Milk may often be a primary cause of poor nutrition in children!"*** This might be due to the fact that proportionate amounts of Vitamins A and D and phosphorus must be present in the metabolism for the proper absorption and utilization of calcium by the body; another reason why proper nutrition and a balanced diet are so important!

Whole milk is a carrier of large amounts of saturated fat (cholesterol) and can lead to atherosclerosis. This food is just for cow's babies. It's wise for humans if they wish to maintain a healthy heart for a long life to eliminate milk!

Calcium Can Help Tame PMS

The mental and physical complaints associated with premenstrual syndrome (PMS) which some women endure monthly prior to menstruation, can be reduced greatly by supplementing with calcium, according to several studies. James G. Penland, Ph.D., a psychologist for U.S. Dept. of Agriculture, placed a group of women with PMS symptoms on a food diet containing 600 mg of calcium. He then gave half the group 700 mg more of calcium in supplement form, and the other half a placebo (sugar pill). Women taking the calcium supplement reported 70% less pain, such as backaches and cramping, and 80% less water retention. **On the emotional side, 90% of women taking the supplement experienced less crying, irritability and depression.** Once again, calcium lived up to its name as "the miracle mineral." A multi-mineral with calcium and magnesium, phosphorus, CoQ10 and 3 mgs of boron is best.

Locations in the Body Where Osteoporosis, Arthritis, Pain and Misery Hit the Hardest

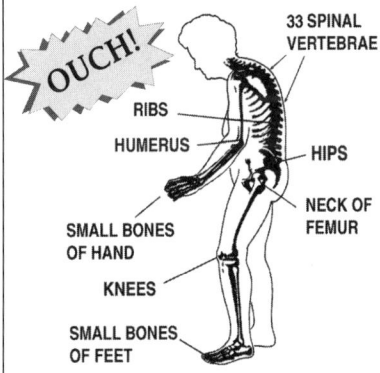

BORON – is an important trace mineral for healthier and stronger bones that also helps the body absorb more vital calcium, minerals and necessary hormones! Good Boron sources are most organic veggies, fresh and sun-dried fruits, avocados, prunes, raw nuts and soybeans.

The U.S. Dept. of Agriculture's Nutrition Lab in Grand Forks, ND, says Boron is usually found in soil and foods, but many Americans eat a diet low in Boron. They conducted a 17 week study which showed a daily 3 to 6 mgs. Boron supplement enabled participants to reduce loss (demineralization) of calcium, phosphorus and magnesium from their bodies. This loss is usually caused by eating processed fast foods, drinking tap waters and eating lots of meat, salt, sugar and fat and a dietary lack of fresh vegetables, fruits and whole grains. (*all-natural.com*)

Scientific studies show women benefit from a healthy lifestyle that includes vitamin D3 sunshine and exercise (even weight lifting) to maintain healthier bones, combined with distilled water, and a diet of low-fat, high-fiber carbohydrates, and fresh organic fruits, salads, sprouts, greens and vegetables. This lifestyle helps protect against heart disease, high blood pressure, cancer and many other ailments! I'm happy to see science now agrees with my Dad who first stated these health truths in the 1920's.

Osteoporosis affects over 52 million & kills 400,000 Americans annually. An estimated 50% of adults 65 years or older suffer from Arthritis.

Some Body Signs of Potassium Deficiency

- Bone and muscle aches and pains, especially lower back.
- The body feels heavy, tired and it's an effort to move.
- Shooting pains when straightening up after leaning over.
- Dizziness upon straightening up after leaning over.
- Morning dull headaches upon arising and when stressed.
- Dull, faded-looking hair that lacks sheen and luster.
- The scalp is itchy and dry. Dandruff, premature hair thinning or balding may occur.
- The hair is unmanageable, mats, often looks straw-like, and is sometimes extremely dry and other times oily.
- The eyes itch, feel sore and uncomfortable and appear bloodshot and watery. Also, eyelids may be granulated with white matter collecting in the corners.

- The eyes tire easily and will not focus as they should.
- You tire physically and mentally with the slightest effort.
- Loss of mental alertness and onset of confusion, making decisions difficult. The memory fails, making you forget familiar names and places you should easily remember.
- You become easily irritable and impatient with family, friends and loved ones and even with your business and social acquaintances.
- You feel nervous, depressed, in a mental fog, and have difficulty getting things done due to mental and muscle fatigue. Even the slightest effort can leave you exhausted, upset and trembling.
- At times, your hands and feet get chilled, even in warm weather, which is a strong sign of potassium deficiency.

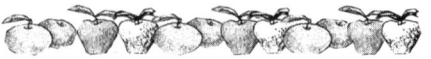

Potassium is necessary for pH balance of your body and for normal blood pressure regulation. Potassium is also needed for muscle growth, your nervous system and brain function. It's found in many different fruits and vegetables. Phytonutrients are also important for health!

Mother Nature's Miracle Phytochemicals Help Prevent Cancer:

Make sure to get your daily dose of naturally occurring, cancer-fighting super foods – Phytonutrients are abundant in apples, tomatoes, onions, garlic, beans, legumes, soybeans, cabbage, cauliflower, broccoli and citrus. Champions with the highest count of Phytonutrients are apples are tomatoes.

Phytonutrient	Food Sources	Health Action
PHYTOESTROGEN ISOFLAVONES	Soy products, flaxseed, seeds and nuts, yams, alfalfa, pomegranates lentils, carrots, apples	Helps block some cancers, aids in menopausal symptoms, balances hormones, helps improve memory, enhances heart health
PHYTOSTEROLS	Plant oils: corn, sesame, safflower; rice bran, wheat germ, peanuts	Blocks hormonal role in cancers, inhibits uptake of cholesterol from diet, reduces risk of heart attack
LIGNANS	Flaxseeds, rye, lentils, soy mushrooms, barley	Helps prevent breast cancer, heart disease and balances hormones
SAPONINS	Yams, beets, beans, cabbage, nuts, soybeans	Helps prevent cancer cells from multiplying, reduces cholesterol
TERPENES	Carrots, winter squash, sweet potatoes, yams, apples, cantaloupes, cherries	Antioxidants – protects DNA from free radical-induced damage, and improves immunity
	Tomatoes and its sauces, tomato-based products	Helps block UVA & UVB and offers help to protect against cancers – breast, prostate, etc.
	Spinach, kale, beet and turnip greens, cabbage	Protects eyes from macular degeneration,
	Red chile peppers	Keeps carcinogens from binding to DNA
QUERCETIN (& FLAVONOIDS)	Apples (especially the skins), red onions and green tea	Strong cancer fighter, protects heart - arteries. Reduces pain, allergy and asthma symptoms
	Citrus fruits (flavonoids)	Promotes protective enzymes
PHENOLS	Apples, fennel, parsley, carrots, alfalfa, cabbage	Helps prevent blood clotting & has important anticancer properties
	Cinnamon	Promotes healthy blood sugar and glucose metabolism
	Citrus fruits, broccoli, cabbage, cucumbers, green peppers, tomatoes	Antioxidants – flavonoids, block membrane receptor sites for certain hormones
	Apples, grape seeds	Strong antioxidants; fights germs and bacteria, strengthens immune system, veins and capillaries
	Grapes, especially skins	Antioxidant, antimutagen; promotes detoxification. Acts as carcinogen inhibitors
	Yellow and green squash	Antihepatotoxic, antitumor
SULFUR COMPOUNDS	Onions and garlic, (fresh is always best) Red onions (our favorite) also contain Quercetin Onions help keep doctor away	Promotes liver enzymes, inhibits cholesterol synthesis, reduces triglycerides, lowers blood pressure improves immune response, fights infections, germs and parasites

Food and Product Summary

Today, many of our foods are highly processed or refined, robbing them of essential nutrients, vitamins, and minerals. Many also contain harmful, toxic and dangerous chemicals. Research findings and experience of top nutritionists, physicians and dentists have led to discoveries that devitalized foods are the major cause of poor health, illness, cancer and premature death! The enormous increase in the last 70 years of degenerative diseases such as heart disease, arthritis, diabetes and dental decay, backs this belief. Scientific research shows most of these afflictions can be prevented and others, once established, can be arrested or even reversed through nutritional methods.

Enjoy Super Health with Natural Foods

1. **RAW FOODS:** Fresh fruits and raw vegetables organically grown are always best! Enjoy a nutritious variety of garden salads with raw vegetables, sprouts, raw nuts and seeds.
2. **VEGETABLES and PROTEINS:**
   a. Legumes, lentils, brown rice, soy beans, and all beans.
   b. Nuts and seeds, raw and unsalted (lightly roasted okay).
   c. We prefer healthier vegetarian proteins. If you must have animal protein, then be sure it's hormone–free, and organically fed and no more than 1 or 2 times a week.
   d. Dairy products – fertile range-free eggs (*not over 4 weekly*), unprocessed hard cheese and feta goat's cheese. We choose not to use dairy products. Try the healthier non-dairy soy, rice, coconut, and almond milks and soy cheeses, delicious soy yogurt and soy and rice ice cream.
3. **FRUITS and VEGETABLES:** Organically grown is always best – grown without the use of poisonous sprays and toxic chemical fertilizers whenever possible; do urge your markets to stock healthier organic produce! Steam, bake, sauté and wok vegetables as short a time as possible to retain the best nutritional content and flavor. Also enjoy fresh juices.
4. **ORGANIC non-GMO WHOLE GRAINS, CEREALS & BREADS:** Barley, rye, buckwheat, spelt, teff, oatmeal, quinoa, millet, amaranth, and wild rice, contain important B-complex vitamins, vitamin E, minerals, fiber and unsaturated fatty acids.
5. **COLD or EXPELLER-PRESSED VEGETABLE OILS:** Organic, first press, extra virgin olive oil (is best), soy, flax, sunflower, and sesame oils are good sources of healthy, essential, unsaturated fatty acids. We still use oils sparingly.

Enjoy Lighter, Smaller Vegetarian Dinners

It seems to be an American custom for people to eat their biggest meal in the evening. From a standpoint of heart attacks, this is the worst time to eat a big meal . . . especially a meal with a preponderance of fat. It has been definitively established by researchers that the blood is more likely to clot 2 to 8 hours following a meal with a high fat intake. It would therefore seem logical to avoid heavy meals – particularly in the evening – to minimize the chances of intravascular clotting. The occurrence of a heart attack after eating a heavy meal has been recognized by doctors for years. Just think of how often you read or hear about a man in his prime dying of a heart attack while in bed at night.

Retired people can regulate their mealtimes easily. Working people can also dine at an earlier hour in the evening and can certainly regulate their diet to promote health and longevity and prolong their golden years!

Light, healthy vegetarian meal is ideal for early evening

It can begin with a raw combination salad (page 109) with an organic healthy dressing followed with 2-3 lightly cooked vegetables – green beans, zucchini, peas, corn, carrots, kale, okra, vegetable stir-fry, etc. Several nights a week add a baked potato – but do not drench this potato in fat! Use organic extra virgin olive oil instead of butter.

We are not telling you that the price you must pay to live a longer life is to give up good flavor. Not at all! The secrets of great flavor are in the use of herbs, garlic, olive oil, onions, green peppers and mushrooms.

A Mediterranean Diet May Alter the Gut Microbiome to Improve Longevity

The Mediterranean Diet – eating fresh vegetables, fruits, whole grains, and fish, as well as drinking a little red wine – is recommended to help improve health and prevent chronic disease. A study published in the journal *Gut* suggests another benefit of the Mediterranean Diet: improving the gut microbiome of older adults and reducing frailty. Your gut microbiome is the community of organisms that live in your intestines that converts many raw food ingredients into beneficial compounds that the body can use.

Avoid These Processed, Refined, Harmful Foods:

Once you realize the harm caused to your body by unhealthy refined, chemicalized, deficient foods, you'll want to eliminate "killer" foods:

- **Refined sugar / artificial sweeteners** (toxic aspartame) or their products such as jams, jellies, preserves, marmalades, yogurts, ice cream, sherbets, Jello, cake, candy, cookies, all chewing gum, colas and diet drinks, pies, pastries, and all sugared fruit juices and fruits canned in sugar syrup. (Health Stores have delicious healthy replacements, such as Stevia, raw honey, 100% maple syrup, and agave nectar, so seek and buy the best).
- **White flour products** such as white bread, wheat-white bread, enriched flours, rye bread that has white flour in it, dumplings, biscuits, buns, gravy, pasta, pancakes, waffles, soda crackers, pizza, ravioli, pies, pastries, cakes, cookies, prepared and commercial puddings and ready-mix bakery products. Most are made with dangerous (oxy-cholesterol) powdered milk and powdered eggs. (Health Stores have a variety of 100% non-GMO whole grain organic products, breads, chips, crackers, pastas, desserts).
- **Salted foods**, such as pretzels, corn chips, potato chips, crackers and nuts.
- **Refined white rice** and pearl barley. • **Fried fast foods.** • **Indian ghee.**
- **Refined dry processed cereals** that are sugared, such as cornflakes, etc.
- **Foods that contain Olestra**, palm and cottonseed oil.
- **Peanuts and peanut butter** that contain hydrogenated, hardened oils and any peanuts with mold and all molds that can cause allergies.
- **Margarine** – combines heart-deadly trans-fatty acids and saturated fats.
- **Saturated fats and hydrogenated oils** – enemies that clog the arteries.
- **Coffee, soft drinks, teas, alcohol, sugared juices** – even if decaffeinated.
- **Fresh pork / products.** • **Fried, fatty, greasy meats.** • **Irradiated GMO foods.**
- **Smoked meats**, such as ham, bacon, sausage and all smoked fish.
- **Luncheon meats**, hot dogs, salami, bologna, corned beef, pastrami and packaged meats containing dangerous sodium nitrate or nitrite.
- **Dried fruits** containing sulphur dioxide – a toxic preservative.
- **Chickens, turkeys and meats injected with hormones** or fed with commercial feed containing any drugs or toxins.
- **Canned soups** – read labels for sugar, salt, starch, flour and preservatives.
- **Foods containing preservatives, additives**, benzoate of soda, salt, sugar, cream of tartar, drugs, irradiated and genetically engineered foods.
- **Day-old cooked vegetables**, potatoes and pre-mixed, wilted lifeless salads.
- **All commercial vinegars:** pasteurized, filtered, distilled, white, malt and synthetic vinegars are dead vinegars! (We use only organic, raw, unfiltered apple cider vinegar with the "Mother Enzyme" as used in olden times.)

Please follow The Bragg Healthy Lifestyle to provide the basic, healthy nourishment to maintain your precious health.

Beware: Why "Modern" Wheat is Bad for You

Modern wheat isn't really wheat at all and is a "perfect, chronic poison," says Dr. William Davis, a Cardiologist, author of *Wheat Belly* Books and a leading expert on wheat, the world's most popular grain. *Dr. Davis explains the wheat we eat today (even though it may say 100% whole wheat), isn't the wheat your ancestors had. It is an 18" tall plant created by genetic research in the 60's and 70's. There's a new protein in this type of wheat called ***gliadin***, which is an opiate. Gliadin binds into opiate receptors in the brain and in most people stimulates appetite – they consume 440 more calories per day, 365 days per year.

Modern wheat is responsible for eight out of ten people's health problems. Researchers have found that once wheat is removed from their diet, their illnesses disappeared within three to six months. People who turn away from wheat have dropped substantial weight. Even diabetics no longer are diabetic; people with arthritis have dramatic relief, along with less acid reflux; leg swelling; irritable bowel syndrome, as well as depression.

So why is wheat bad? Wheat is one of the oldest known grains. When grown in organic, fertile soil, non-GMO whole wheat is rich in vitamins E and B complex, many minerals, including calcium and iron, as well as omega-3 fatty acids.

Unfortunately, the modern version of wheat is a far cry from these ancient plants. As with other commercially grown grains, scientists began cross-breeding wheat plants to arrive at new varieties that are hardier, shorter, and yield more. In fact, the newer, high-yield hybridized wheat we've been eating since the 1980's has been selectively bred to produce high gluten grains that seem to trigger inflammatory responses in our body, causing more problems than ever! Among the diseases attributed to the consumption of wheat is Celiac disease.

Dr. Davis says "that there is no nutrient deficiency that develops when eliminating wheat from your diet. Replace wheat with organic healthy foods like vegetables; nuts, avocados. Try eliminating grains, that's when you will see transformations in your health." *See *IntentionalWellnessInc.com/nutrition/wheat-is-bad-for-you*

Keep Blood Sugar Levels Low and Healthy

Australian researcher and one of the authors of *The Glucose Revolution,* Dr. Jennie Brand-Miller cites in her book, that when you eat carbohydrates – any sugary or starchy food – your blood sugar goes up! If it rises slowly, that's ideal; however, if it soars quickly, this could lead to serious health threats. Researchers at Harvard Medical School have also cited that a spike in blood sugar can double or triple your risk of developing Type 2 (adult onset) diabetes.

Dr. Brand-Miller has created a Glycemic Index (GI) that ranks foods based on how quickly they raise blood sugar. Several factors influence the glycemic index of a food, including its nutrient composition, cooking method, ripeness, and the amount of processing it has undergone. High-glycemic-index foods (70 or higher) make blood sugar jump quickly; Low-glycemic-index foods (55 or less) cause a slower rise.

- Eat health giving legumes such as lentils, soybeans, lima and kidney beans, black beans, chick peas, etc., for they promote a gradual blood sugar rise and have a low-glycemic index.
- Eating organic brown rice, lentils, quinoa, couscous, and non-starchy vegetables: broccoli, cauliflower and spinach, are healthy, filling and they help normalize blood sugar and reduce appetite that helps in weight loss.
- If you snack, choose fresh organic fruits, even popcorn.
- Eat fresh, organic vegetables. Think of salad vegetables as "free" foods, with no significant impact on blood sugar or weight. It's best to avoid fatty foods, sugars, and meat.
- Avoid all processed, refined foods: refined breads, cereals, cookies, crackers, and desserts. These refined starches zip through your digestive tract, raising your blood sugar.

***EATING APPLES CAN GIVE YOU A BURST OF ENERGY:** Not only will an apple a day keep the doctor away, it'll also give you a powerful jolt of energy. Apples are high in fiber, so they take longer to digest. Snack on apples for an effective pick-me-up. Also, researchers found a significant boost in endurance capacity from the quercetin in red apples. Quercetin is a natural antioxidant that boosts the power of the mitochondria (the powerhouse of the cell) in your muscles and brain; this surge of power gives you energy!*

Increase Your Stamina and Go Power

If you eat right you will be able to go the distance, whether it's competing in a triathlon or the next sports marathon work day. It is important to boost stamina by taking advantage of the way energy is released in the body and trying to keep this process from getting bogged down. The body breaks food down into blood sugar, or glucose, which powers the cells. Nutrients such as B vitamins, iron, magnesium and zinc play vital roles in driving this energy-providing process. It's crucial to increasing and maintaining your stamina that you get enough of them. Overindulging in nutrient-rich food can be counterproductive, if the body expends too much energy digesting food that's not immediately needed, then precious energy is wasted.

Stamina – Boosting Foods and Nutrients

- Kidney beans and lentils • Water – purified, distilled
- Organic grains, pastas, oatmeal, cereals, barley, brown rice
- Spinach, swiss chard, kale and other leafy greens

Vitamins and minerals, which play important roles in all of the chemical processes of the body, help maintain stamina in two primary ways: helping your body break down the high-energy foods you eat and use as energy; and helping your brain produce chemicals that make you feel energetic for a sustained period. A few of the most important nutrients when it comes to stamina are: iron, 18-30 mgs. daily; calcium, 250-800 mgs. daily; and magnesium, 125-400 mgs. daily. (See page 122.)

The Stamina Balance

Nutritionists recommend you get 55 to 60% of calories from complex carbohydrates like non-GMO whole-grain bread, cereal, rice, grains and pasta. These provide a slow, steady release of energy and also contain the vitamins and minerals you need to produce energy. Athletes take advantage of this time-released energizing power by "carbo-loading." Balancing carbs with protein-rich foods like beans works well for the normal person.

The purpose of life is a life of purpose. – Robert Byrne

Boost Your Memory

The mental function of memory allows us to recall ideas, facts, sensations and impressions. There are three types of memory: sensory, short-term and long-term. We never really give memory much thought until we forget where we parked the car or forget an appointment or have trouble remembering a name. There are many factors which affect the memory, such as your overall health, diet, age, hormone levels and some medications. However there are several things you can do to preserve or improve your memory. Scientists are discovering nutrients found in certain foods help enhance the memory and they are easy to include in your meals.

The Brain – Memory Boosting Diet

Consuming a low-fat diet to keep cholesterol in check is the very first step you should take toward improving your memory. This is vital because high cholesterol levels inhibit the flow of oxygen to your brain and cause the memory to falter. The next step is simply to add foods to your diet that benefit brain and nerve function. One serving of grains, soy, brown rice or lentils and five servings of organic fruits and vegetables provide nutrients needed to bolster your memory. Certain lifestyle changes that enhance memory are to avoid second-hand smoke and NEVER smoke, or use recreational drugs or alcohol!

Nutrients and Herbs to the Rescue

Ginkgo biloba, ginseng, and rosemary have been used for thousands of years to enhance memory. Studies show that these herbs have antioxidant properties that aid blood and oxygen flow to the brain. Ginkgo also helps boost metabolism and electrical brain activity. Rosemary, known as "the remembrance herb," helps prevent the breakdown of acetylcholine, a brain chemical crucial to memory. Also try Niacin (B3 – 100mg) daily with meal.

Whole grains and fish oils help boost memory. Also try beets, blueberries, turmeric, broccoli, dark chocolate, oranges, and the phytoestrogens in yams, flaxseeds, raw nuts and seeds also help improve memory (page 91).

CROSS-TRAIN YOUR BRAIN: keep it youthful – brain exchange with family, friends, chat groups and learn new challenges, games, dancing, gardening.

Plant-Based Protein Chart

BEANS & LEGUMES

(1 cup cooked)	PROTEIN IN GRAMS
Soybeans	29
Lentils	18
Adzuki Beans	17
Cannellini	17
Navy Beans	16
Split Peas	16
Black Beans	15
Garbanzos (chick peas)	15
Kidney Beans	15
Great Northern Beans	15
Lima Beans	15
Black-eyed Peas	14
Pinto Beans	14
Mung Beans	14
Tofu (3 oz.)	7 to 12
Green Peas (whole)	9

RAW NUTS & SEEDS

(1/4 cup or 4 Tbsps)	PROTEIN IN GRAMS
Chia Seeds	12
Macadamia Nuts	11
Flax Seeds	8
Sunflower Seeds	8
Almonds	7
Pumpkin Seeds	7
Sesame Seeds	7
Walnuts	5
Brazil Nuts	5
Hazelnuts	5
Pine Nuts	4
Cashews	4

NUT BUTTERS

(2 Tbsps)	PROTEIN IN GRAMS
Peanut Butter	7 to 9
Almond Butter	5 to 8
Cashew Butter	4 to 5
Sesame - Tahini	6

VEGETABLES

(1 Serving or 1 cup)	PROTEIN IN GRAMS
Spirulina	8.6
Corn (1 cob)	5
Potato (with skin)	5
Mushrooms, Oyster	5
Artichoke (1 medium)	4
Collard Greens	4
Broccoli	4
Brussel Sprouts	4
Mushrooms, Shitake	3.5
Swiss Chard	3
Kale	2.5
Asparagus (5 spears)	2
String Beans	2
Beets	2
Peas	2
Sweet Potato	3
Summer Squash	2
Cabbage	2
Carrot	2
Cauliflower	2
Squash	2
Celery	1
Spinach	1
Bell Peppers	1
Cucumber	1
Eggplant	1
Leeks	1
Lettuce	1
Tomato (1 medium)	1
Radish	1
Turnips	1

DAIRY & NUT MILKS

(1 cup)	PROTEIN IN GRAMS
Oat Milk	3 to 4
Almond Milk	1 to 2
Rice Milk	1
Eggs (1) *(free-range)*	6

FRUITS

(1 Serving or 1 cup)	PROTEIN IN GRAMS
Avocado (1 medium)	4
Banana (1)	1 to 2
Blackberries (1 cup)	2
Pomegranate (1)	1.5
Blueberries (1 cup)	1
Cantaloupe (1 cup)	1
Cherries (1 cup)	1
Grapes (1 cup)	1
Honeydew (1 cup)	1
Kiwi (1 large)	1
Lemon (1)	1
Mango (1)	1
Nectarine (1)	1
Orange (1)	1
Peach (1)	1
Pear (1)	1
Pineapple (1 cup)	1
Plum (1)	1
Raspberries (1 cup)	1
Strawberries (1 cup)	1
Watermelon (1 cup)	1

GRAINS & RICE

(1 cup cooked)	PROTEIN IN GRAMS
Triticale	25
Millet	8.4
Amaranth	7
Oat Bran	7
Wild Rice	7
Couscous (whole wheat)	6
Bulgar Wheat	6
Buckwheat	6
Teff	6
Oat Groats	6
Barley	5
Quinoa	5
Brown Rice	5
Spelt	5

This chart displays protein content of common vegetarian foods.

Note that in order to determine amount of protein that is optimal for your body, use the following formula that is based on a vegan diet: *RDA recommends that we take in 0.36 grams of protein per pound that we weigh* (100 lbs. x 0.36 = 36 grams).

Data from webs: *TheHolyKale.com • VegParadise.com • vrg.org (Vegetarian Resource Group).*

Vegetable and Fruit Juices Contain Mother Nature's Distilled Water

No new water has been put on the face of Mother Earth since it was originally formed. Just as the same energy is formed and re-formed, so the same water is used and re-used over and over again by the miracle of Mother Nature. Waters of the earth are purified by distillation. The sun evaporates the water which is collected into clouds. When the clouds become full we have rain and dew – pure, perfectly clean, distilled water, free of all harmful inorganic substances, until polluted!

Years ago, when the late Douglas Fairbanks Sr. and Dad were close friends, they roamed the South Sea Islands for several months. During that trip Dad came upon an island inhabited by *beautiful, healthy Polynesians* who drank only distilled rain water because the island was surrounded by the Pacific Ocean. Their island was based on porous coral which could not hold water – so they would *only drink rain water* or the fresh, clear, clean water of the green coconut. (Rain water is stored worldwide by millions.) Dad had never seen any finer specimens of humanity than these native South Sea Islanders. There were several doctors on the yacht who thoroughly examined the most mature people on these islands. One heart doctor stated that he had never in his life examined such healthy, well-preserved people.

You may have noted we said only the most mature people were examined by the doctors. *They were so completely unaware of age* that no such word existed in their language! They never celebrated birthdays, so they were forever young – gloriously ageless, not only in years but in body. These older men performed as well in the vigorous native dances as the younger men. **They were all beautiful human specimens because they lived their lengthy lives drinking only pure distilled water, eating natural foods and enjoying a happy, healthy lifestyle.**

I now live on legumes, vegetables and fruits. No dairy, no meat of any kind, no chicken, no turkey, and very little fish, only once in a while. It changed my metabolism and I lost 24 pounds. I did research and found 82% of people who go on a plant-based diet begin to heal themselves, as I did.

– Bill Clinton, United States President, 1993-2001

Chart is from book: Water – The Shocking Truth, see back pages for booklist.

The 75% Watery Human

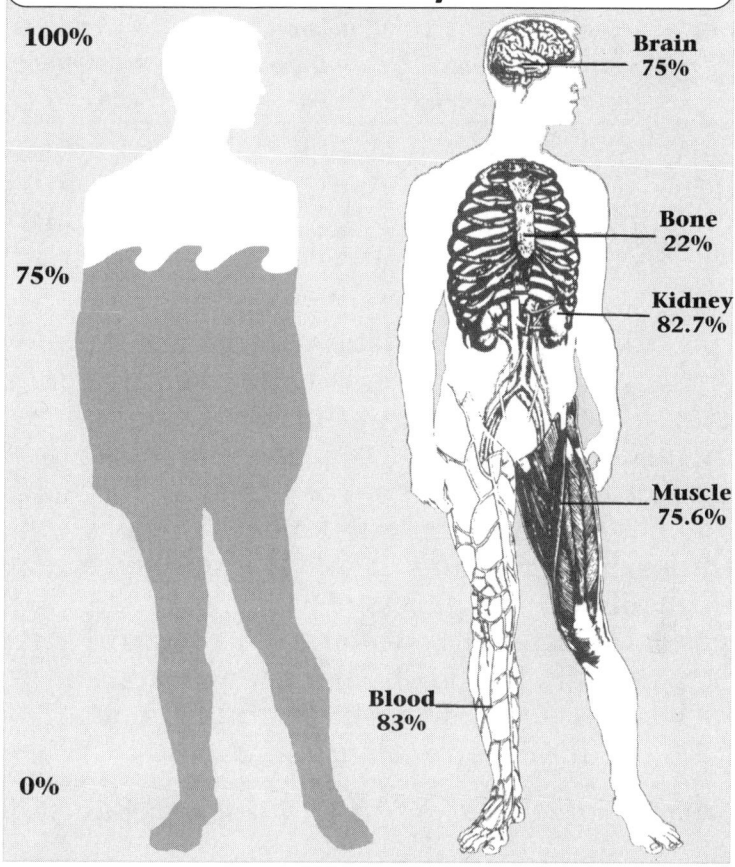

The amount of water in the human body averages 60%, but can vary considerably from one part of the body to another as shown here. A lean man may hold 75% of his weight in body water, while a woman – because of her larger proportion of water-poor fatty tissues – may be only 52% water. The lowering of the water content in the blood is what triggers the hypothalamus, the brain's vital thirst center, to send out its familiar urgent demand for a drink of water! Please obey and drink ample amounts (8 glasses) of purified, distilled water daily. By the time you feel thirsty, you're already dehydrated. – American Running & Fitness Association

WATER PERCENTAGE IN VARIOUS BODY PARTS:

Teeth	*10%*	*Spleen*	*75.5%*
Bones	*22%*	*Lungs*	*80%*
Cartilage	*55%*	*Blood*	*83%*
Red blood corpuscles	*68.7%*	*Bile*	*86%*
Liver	*71.5%*	*Plasma*	*90%*
Brain	*75%*	*Lymph*	*94%*
Muscle tissue	*75%*	*Saliva*	*95.5%*

This chart shows why 8-10 glasses of pure water daily is so important.

Water is the Key to All Body Functions:

- *Heart*
- *Glands*
- *Sex*
- *Muscles*
- *Metabolism*
- *Bones & Joints*
- *Energy*
- *Digestion*
- *Elimination*
- *Circulation*
- *Assimilation*
- *Nerves*

The body is 75% water and pure, steam-distilled (chemical-free) water is important for total health. You should drink at least 8 glasses of water daily. Read our book, *Water – The Shocking Truth*, for more info on the importance of pure water. See back pages for booklist.

Pure, distilled water is vitally important in following The Bragg Healthy Lifestyle. Water is the key to all body functions including: digestion, circulation, bones and joints, assimilation, elimination, muscles, nerves, glands, sex and senses. The right kind of water is one of your best natural protections against all kinds of diseases and viral infections, such as influenza and pneumonia. It is a vital factor in all body fluids, tissues, cells, lymph, blood and all glandular secretions. Water holds all nutritive factors in solution, as well as toxins and body wastes, and acts as the main transportation medium throughout the body, for both nutritional and cleansing purposes!

Distilled Water is the World's Purest and Best Water!

It's excellent for detoxification, fasting and cleansing of cells, organs and body fluids, because it helps carry away harmful toxins and substances (purified and reverse osmosis water is acceptable also). Water from all chemically treated public water systems – and even from many wells and springs – is likely to be loaded with poisonous chemicals and toxic trace elements. Depending upon the kinds of pipes used in the buildings, the water is likely to be overloaded with lead (from older, soldered pipe joints), zinc (from old-fashioned galvanized pipes) or with copper and cadmium (from copper pipes). These trace elements are released in dangerous quantities by the chemical action of the water flowing against the metals of the pipes.

"Distilled water plays a vital part in treatment of illness, arthritis, etc."
– Dr. Allen Banik in his book, "The Choice is Clear"

There is only one water that is purified clean and that is steam distilled water. No other substance on our planet does so much to keep us healthy and get us well as this water does. – Dr. James Balch, author of "Prescription for Dietary Wellness"

Allergies & Dr. Coca's Pulse Test

Almost every known food may cause some allergic reaction at times. Thus, foods used in elimination diets may cause allergic reactions in some individuals. Some are listed among the Most Common Food Allergies (see below). Since reaction to these foods is generally low, they are widely used in making test diets. By keeping a food journal and tracking your pulse rate after meals you will soon know your problem foods. Allergenic foods cause your pulse to then go up. (Take base pulse, for 1 minute, before meals, then 30 minutes after meals, and also before bed. If it increases 8-10 beats per minute – check foods for allergies.)

If your body has a reaction after eating some particular food, especially if it happens each time you eat that food, you may have an allergy. Some allergic reactions are: wheezing, sneezing, stuffy nose, nasal drip or mucus, dark circles, eye watering or bags under your eyes, headaches, feeling light-headed or dizzy, fast heart beat, stomach or chest pains, diarrhea, extreme thirst, breaking out in a rash, swelling of extremities or stomach bloating. Do read Dr. Arthur Coca's book, *The Pulse Test.*

If you know what you're allergic to, you are lucky; if you don't, you had better find out as fast as possible and eliminate all irritating foods from your diet. To re-evaluate your daily life and have a health guide to your future, start a daily journal (keep an 8 ½ x 11 notebook – enlarge and copy form on next page) of foods eaten, your pulse rate before and after meals and your reactions, moods, energy levels, weight, elimination and sleep patterns. You will discover the foods and situations causing problems. By charting your diet you will be amazed at the effects of eating certain foods. We have kept daily journals for years.

If you are hypersensitive to certain foods, you must omit them from your diet! There are hundreds of allergies and of course it's impossible here to take up each one. Many have allergies to milk, wheat, or some are allergic to all grains. Visit web: *FoodAllergy.org.* Your daily journal will help you discover and accurately pinpoint the foods and situations causing you problems. Start your journal today!

Most Common Food Allergies

- **DAIRY:** Butter, Cheese, Cottage Cheese, Ice Cream, Milk, Yogurt, etc.
- **CEREALS & GRAINS:** Wheat, Corn, Buckwheat, Oats, Rye
- **EGGS:** Cakes, Custards, Dressings, Mayonnaise, Noodles
- **FISH:** Shellfish, Crabs, Lobster, Shrimp, Shad Roe
- **MEATS:** Bacon, Beef, Chicken, Pork, Sausage, Veal, Smoked Products
- **FRUITS:** Citrus Fruits, Melons, Strawberries
- **NUTS:** Peanuts, Pecans, Walnuts, chemically dried preserved nuts
- **MISCELLANEOUS:** Chocolate, Cocoa, Coffee, Black & Green (caffeine) Teas, Palm & Cottonseed Oils, MSG & Salt.

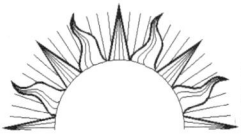

Enlarge and copy this journal page to use in a 3 ring binder.

MY DAILY HEALTH JOURNAL

Today is:____/____/____

I have said my morning resolve and am ready to practice faithfully The Bragg Healthy Lifestyle today and every day.

Yesterday I went to bed at: Today I arose at: Weight:

Today I practiced the No-Heavy Breakfast or No-Breakfast Plan: ☐ yes ☐ no

- For Breakfast I drank: Time:

  For Breakfast I ate:

  Time:

  Supplements:

- For Lunch I ate: Time:

  Supplements:

- For Dinner I ate: Time:

  Supplements:

- ____ Glasses of Water I Drank during the Day, including ACV Drinks

  List Snacks – Kind and When:

- I took part in these physical activities (walking, gym, etc.) today:

Grade each on scale of 1 to 10 (desired optimum health is 10).

- I rate my day for the following categories:

Previous Night's Sleep:	Stress/Anxiety:
Energy Level:	Elimination:
Physical Activity, Exercise:	Health:
Peacefulness:	Accomplishments:
Happiness:	Self-Esteem:

- General Comments, Reactions and any To-Do List:

Dr. Charles Attwood – Great Health Crusader

As a doctor, humanitarian, strong dedicated Health Crusader and a devoted Pediatrician for over 40 years, and Fellow of the American Academy of Pediatrics, Dr. Charles Raymond Attwood fought many battles against mainstream medicine and big business to ensure the health of people everywhere, particularly children. He championed a low-fat vegetarian menu for children, was a strong health and nutrition activist and an associate of Dr. Benjamin Spock. One major battle occurred in 1996. As a member of the Center for Science in the Public Interest, Dr. Attwood led opposition to the giant Gerber Baby Food Company's practice of diluting its baby foods with water, sugar and starch! He won! Gerber stopped this 40 year crime against America's children. Now their foods are 100% fruits and vegetables. Other baby food companies then followed. *VegSource.com.*

Dr. Attwood held high the banner advocating a low-fat, plant-based diet as the most healthy for youngsters. His highly praised 1995 book, *Dr. Attwood's Low-Fat Prescription for Kids* makes a strong scientific argument for this diet. His research shows to avoid the leading causes of premature death later as adults: heart disease, stroke, cancers, diabetes, etc. it's important children follow his program.

Dr. Attwood's Tips for Low-Fat Shopping

- Spend most of your time in the produce department.
- Try new varieties of produce. Look at those with the most intense colors and remember organic is best!
- Don't forget about pasta made from whole-grains.
- Go straight for the whole-grain breads section.
- Buy unrefined, low-fat, sugarless, high-fiber cereals.
- When buying packaged, canned, frozen foods, read labels.
- Don't underestimate beans – whether dried, frozen or canned, they are delicious and healthy for you.
- Buy low- or no-fat healthy snacks – there are many choices. Careful as some are high in salt, sugar and calories.
- Replace milk and low-fat dairy products with soy, nut, coconut, rice milks, and soy, tofu cheeses, etc.

Dr. Kellogg's Famous Menus:

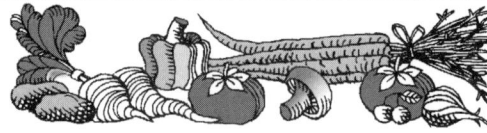

Menu #1

Breakfast

Organic natural sun-dried apricots* topped with raw wheat germ and
sliced banana, pear or orange (if desired)
(*soak in jar overnight in distilled water or unsweetened pineapple juice)
OR
you may substitute the
Bragg Healthy Energy Smoothie Drink on page 108 for a delicious energy breakfast. Remember to earn your breakfast by engaging in some exercise first.

Lunch

Organic Raw Vegetable Combination Salad
grated raw beet, carrot, turnip, zucchini, chopped tomato, cabbage, green onions and sprouts: alfalfa, mung or sunflower

For dressing mix apple cider vinegar (or lemon juice), organic extra-virgin olive oil (or try flaxseed or hempseed oil) and garlic with a dab of raw honey

1/4 cup of raw sunflower or pumpkin seeds (rich in protein and natural oil)

Raw apple

Dinner

Organic Green-Leaf Variety Salad
with raw mixed lettuces and spinach, kale, cucumber, carrot, celery, tomato, parsley or watercress

Protein – tofu or cooked brown rice with beans or lentils *(Recipe on page 109)*

Fresh fruit

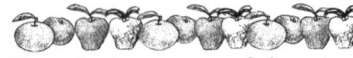

Apples give you Vitamin C – a powerful antioxidant and pectin, a soluble fiber that can help lower cholesterol and glucose (sugar) levels!

Dr. Kellogg's Famous Menus:

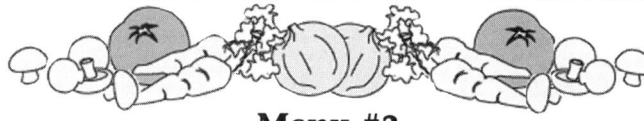

Menu #2

Breakfast

Apple sauce*
Steel cut oats– hot cereal**
served with honey, blackstrap molasses,
pure maple syrup or stevia
100% whole wheat or rye toast
(*Make your own apple sauce, if desired add honey)
(**Top and serve with sliced ripe banana or other fruit)

Lunch

Organic Raw Vegetable Combination Salad
(Same as 1st day)
Vegetable soup with natural barley and lentils
whole rye toast or oat bran-raisin muffin

Dinner

Cabbage, apple & carrot coleslaw
with spring onions
brown rice or baked potato with skin
baked or steamed carrots and peas
fresh fruit
OR
Avocado, red onion and tomato salad
steamed asparagus or broccoli
raw nuts and seeds of any kind
Fresh fruit

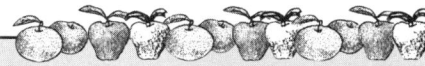

Eat Plenty of Cabbage: A Miracle Cleanser & Healer

Raw cabbage has amazing properties. It stimulates your immune system, kills bacteria and viruses, and helps heal ulcers. According to Dr. James Balch in *Prescription for Cooking and Dietary Wellness*, your chances of contracting colon cancer can be reduced by up to 60% by eating cabbage weekly. Therapeutic benefits have also been attributed to cabbage in relation to scurvy, gout, rheumatism arthritis, eye diseases, asthma, pyorrhea and gangrene. We love raw cabbage and also make a variety of sandwiches wrapped in cabbage leaves instead of bread.

HEALTHY BEVERAGES
Fresh Juices, Herb Teas & Energy Drinks

These freshly squeezed organic vegetable and fruit juices are important to *The Bragg Healthy Lifestyle*. It's not wise to drink beverages with your main meals, as it dilutes the digestive juices. But it's great during the day to have a glass of freshly squeezed orange juice, grapefruit juice, vegetable juice, raw, organic apple cider vinegar drink (see below), or herbal tea – these are all ideal pick-me-up beverages.

Apple Cider Vinegar Drink – Mix 1-2 tsps. raw, organic apple cider vinegar (with the 'Mother' enzyme) and (optional) to taste raw honey or pure maple syrup *(if diabetic, to sweeten use 2 stevia drops)* in 8 oz. of distilled or purified water. Take glass upon arising, an hour before lunch and dinner.

Delicious Hot or Cold Cider Drink – Add 2-3 cinnamon sticks and 4 cloves to water and boil. Steep 20 minutes or more. Before serving add raw organic apple cider vinegar and sweetener to taste.

Bragg's Favorite Juice Drink – This drink consists of all raw vegetables *(remember organic is best)* which we prepare in our juicer / blender: carrots, celery, cucumber, beets, cabbage, tomatoes, watercress, kale, parsley, or any vegetable combination you prefer. The great purifier, garlic we enjoy, but it's optional.

Bragg's Favorite Healthy Energy Smoothie – After our morning stretch and exercises we often enjoy the drink below instead of fruit. It's a delicious and powerfully nutritious meal anytime: lunch, dinner or in a thermos at work, school, sports, the gym and during sports or hikes. You can freeze for popsicles too.

Bragg's Favorite Healthy Energy Smoothie

Prepare the following in a blender, add frozen juice cubes if desired colder; Choice of: freshly squeezed orange or grapefruit juice; carrot and greens juice; unsweetened pineapple juice; or 1 1/2 - 2 cups purified or distilled water with:

2 tsps spirulina or green powder
1/3 tsp Nutritional Yeast
2 dates or prunes-pitted
1 tsp protein powder (optional)

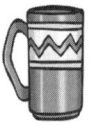

1-2 bananas or fresh fruit
1-2 tsps almond or nut butter
1 tsp flaxseed oil or grind seeds
1 tsp raw honey (optional)

Optional: 4-6 apricots (sun-dried,) soak in jar overnight in purified water or unsweetened pineapple juice. We soak enough to last for several days. Keep refrigerated. In summer you can add organic fresh fruit: peaches, papaya, blueberries, strawberries, all berries, apricots, etc. instead of banana. In winter, add apples, kiwi, oranges, tangelos, persimmons or pears, and if fresh is unavailable, try sugar-free, frozen organic fruits. Serves 1 to 2.

Patricia's Delicious Health Popcorn

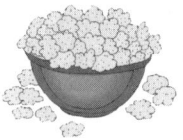

Use freshly popped organic popcorn (use air popper). Drizzle organic olive oil, melted coconut oil or salt-free butter over popcorn. Sprinkle with good quality nutritional yeast for amazing flavor. For a variety try a pinch of cayenne pepper, mustard powder or fresh crushed garlic to oil mixture. Serve instead of breads!

Healthy, healing dietary fibers are organic fresh vegetables, fruits, salads whole grains and their products. These health builders help normalize your blood pressure, cholesterol and promotes healthy elimination

Lentil & Brown Rice Casserole, Burgers or Soup
Paul Bragg and Jack LaLanne's Favorite Recipe

16 oz pkg organic lentils, uncooked
1 cup brown organic rice, uncooked
5 cups, distilled / purified water
4-6 carrots, chop 1/2" rounds
3 celery stalks, chop
4 garlic cloves, chop
2 onions, chop
2 tsps organic coconut aminos
1 tsp salt-free all-purpose seasoning
2 tsps organic extra-virgin olive oil
1 cup diced fresh or canned tomatoes (salt-free)

Wash and drain lentils and rice. Place grains in large stainless steel pot. Add water, bring to boil, reduce heat and simmer 30 minutes. Now add vegetables and seasonings and cook on low heat until tender. Last five minutes add fresh or canned (salt-free) tomatoes. For delicious garnish, add minced parsley. **For Burgers mash. For Soup, add more water in cooking grains.** Serves 4 to 6.

Patricia's Raw Organic Vegetable Health Salad

2 stalks celery, chop
1 bell pepper & seeds, dice
1/2 cucumber, slice
2 carrots, grate
1 raw beet, grate
1 cup green cabbage, chop
1/2 cup red cabbage, chop
1/2 cup alfalfa, mung or sunflower sprouts
2 spring onions & green tops, chop
1 turnip, grate
1 avocado (ripe)
3 tomatoes, medium size

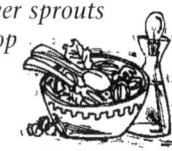

For variety add organic raw zucchini, peas, mushrooms, broccoli, cauliflower, (try black olives and pasta). Chop, slice or grate vegetables fine to medium for variety in size. Mix vegetables & serve on bed of lettuce, spinach, chopped kale or cabbage. Dice avocado and tomato and serve on side as a dressing. Serve choice of fresh squeezed lemon, orange or dressing separately. Chill salad plates before serving. **It's best to always eat salad first before hot dishes.** Serves 3 to 5.

Patricia's Health Salad Dressing

1/2 cup raw organic apple cider vinegar
1-2 tsps organic raw honey
1/2 tsp organic coconut aminos
1-2 cloves garlic, minced
1/3 cup organic extra-virgin olive oil, or blend with safflower, soy, sesame or flax oil
1 Tbsp fresh herbs, minced (to taste)

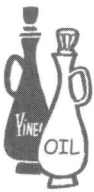

Blend ingredients in blender or jar. Refrigerate in covered jar.

For delicious Herbal Vinegar: In quart jar add 1/3 cup tightly packed, crushed fresh sweet basil, tarragon, dill, oregano, or any fresh herbs desired, combined or singly (If dried herbs, use 1-2 tsps herbs). Now cover to top with raw, organic apple cider vinegar and store two weeks in warm place, and then strain and refrigerate.

Honey – Chia or Celery Seed Vinaigrette

1/4 tsp dry mustard
1/4 tsp organic coconut aminos
1/4 tsp paprika or to taste
1-2 Tbsps honey
1 cup organic apple cider vinegar
1/2 cup organic extra-virgin olive oil
1/2 small onion, minced
1/3 tsp chia or celery seed (or vary to taste)

Blend ingredients in blender or jar. Refrigerate in covered jar.

Studies show both beta carotene and vitamin C, abundantly found in fruits and vegetables, play vital roles in preventing heart disease and cancers.

BENEFITS FROM THE JOYS OF FASTING

Fasting renews your faith in yourself, your strength and God's strength.
Fasting is easier than any diet.
Fasting is the quickest way to lose weight.
Fasting is adaptable to a busy life.
Fasting gives the body a physiological rest.
Fasting is used successfully in the treatment of many physical illnesses.
Fasting can yield weight losses of up to 10 pounds or more in the first week.
Fasting lowers and normalizes cholesterol, homocysteine, blood pressure levels.
Fasting improves dietary habits.
Fasting increases pleasure eating healthy foods.
Fasting is a calming experience, often relieving tension and insomnia.
Fasting frequently induces feelings of happy euphoria, a natural high.
Fasting is a miracle rejuvenator, helps in slowing the ageing process.
Fasting is a natural stimulant to rejuvenate the growth hormone levels.
Fasting is an energizer, not a debilitator.
Fasting aids the elimination process.
Fasting often results in a more vigorous happy marital relationship.
Fasting can eliminate smoking, drug and drinking addictions.
Fasting is a regulator, educating the body to consume food only as needed.
Fasting saves precious time spent on marketing, preparing and eating.
Fasting rids the body of toxins, giving it an internal shower and cleansing.
Fasting does not deprive the body of essential nutrients.
Fasting can be used to uncover the sources of food allergies.
Fasting is used effectively in schizophrenia and other mental illness treatment.
Fasting under proper supervision can be tolerated easily up to four weeks.
Fasting does not accumulate appetite; hunger pangs disappear in 1-2 days.
Fasting is routine for most of the animal kingdom.
Fasting has been a common practice since the beginning of man's existence.
Fasting is practiced in all religions; the Bible alone has 74 references to fasting.
Fasting under proper conditions is absolutely safe.
Fasting is a blessing – "Fasting As A Way Of Life" – Allan Cott, M.D.
Fasting is not starving, it's nature's cure that God has given us. – Patricia Bragg

Dear Health Friend,

This gentle reminder explains the great benefits from "The Miracle of Fasting" that you will enjoy when starting on your weekly 24-hour Bragg Fasting Program for Super Health! It's a precious time of body-mind-soul cleansing and renewal.

On fast days I drink 8-10 glasses of distilled (our favorite) or purified water, (I add 1-2 tsps. organic apple cider vinegar to three of them). If just starting, you may also try herbal teas or try diluted fresh juices with 1/3 distilled water. Every day, even on fast days, add 1 Tbsp. of psyllium husk powder to liquids once daily. It's an extra cleanser and helps normalize weight, cholesterol and blood pressure and helps promote healthy elimination. Fasting is the oldest, most effective healing method known to man. Fasting offers great miraculous blessings from Mother Nature and our Creator. It begins the self-cleansing of the inner-body workings so we can promote our own self-healing.

My father and I wrote the book "The Miracle of Fasting" to share with you the health miracles it can perform in your life. It's all so worthwhile to do. It's an important part of The Bragg Healthy Lifestyle.

With Love, Patricia

Paul Bragg's work on fasting and water is one of the great contributions to the healing wisdom and the natural health movement in the world today. – Gabriel Cousens, M.D., author "Conscious Eating" and "Spiritual Nutrition"

Exercise Your Body

Fourth Step Towards Building Nerve Force

There is nothing better to build powerful Nerve Force than a brisk two to five mile hike everyday. You're too old and flabby? Nonsense! Dad was a great-great-grandfather and he loved to hike, jog, run, swim, ride his bicycle, climb mountains, play tennis and enjoyed playing many other athletic sports. You're never too old to start! Of course, we don't expect you to plunge right in and become an athlete overnight! Do it gradually. Start out with a one mile hike every day for a week. Then increase it to two miles. As you exercise your muscles, your blood starts circulating briskly through your body. Breathe deeply and fill your lungs with more oxygen. You will then feel new vigor and vitality surging through you! You will eat with a good appetite and you will sleep like a baby. **Your Nerve Force reservoirs will soon be filled with energy, go-power and you will have a new zest for living!**

The more time you spend in the fresh air and gentle sunshine doing physical activity, the greater your reserves of Nerve Force will be! In our long experience as teachers of health, fitness and longevity, we found those who exercise regularly have greater poise and a more balanced personality. They are also generally free from nervous and emotional stress that plague the typically inactive person.

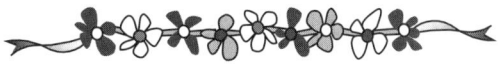

Exercising 15-30 minutes or more a day helps to maintain healthy blood vessels for good circulation in the body and brain and helps you manage your weight and stress levels. Studies have shown that brisk walking helps delay brain shrinkage that delays the onset of dementia.

Exercise, aerobics, walking, biking, roller-blading, swimming, jogging, tennis and most all sports benefit your body and brain power and help you think faster. Studies show exercise keeps the brain younger and helps to retain the quick response of youth.

A good laugh, a good walk and a good sleep are the best cures in the doctor's book!

In the Hawaiian Islands, swimming is so ideal that Hawaii has had great fun hosting swimming contests with youngsters of all ages. They splash and dive in the water, and their merry laughter would ring in the clear, tropical air! When we would talk to parents of these active children, we found they had absolutely no emotional or social problems with them. No matter what your age, exercise can do wonders for you! It's never too late to start tapping the rich veins of vitality lying dormant within every person! If you want to be well-balanced emotionally and free of stresses, strains and tensions – make it a habit to get outdoors for physical activity at least once every day.

Walking Helps Remove Emotional Tensions

We learned many years ago that we could actually walk off our emotional stress. No matter how serious the problems we faced, we could find the answer to our dilemma in a brisk two mile walk. Some of the greatest decisions we have had to make in our lives were made during one of our hikes. As the oxygen floods into the body from vigorous walking, one can think more clearly.

A wealthy friend telephoned Dad during the great financial depression of the 1930s and said, "Paul, I am completely ruined financially. I am going to kill myself, and I called up to say good-bye." My father asked this tormented man to grant him just one favor. When he agreed, Dad said, "All right, we will have a walk in the great outdoors and a farewell talk before you end your life."

Dad got in his car, dashed to his friend's home and off they went, hiking for a full five hours. During that time father told him that money was not the only thing in life and that he had to get some perspective and straighten out his values. Dad literally walked some sense into him! Had that man stayed at home and brooded over his loses, he would have destroyed himself and family. That long nature walk in fresh air changed his whole life! Dad's friend was not rich materially, but rich in inner wealth.

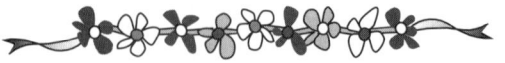

If I had to pick one thing . . . that comes closest to the Fountain of Youth, it would be exercise!

– Dr. James Fries, M.D., expert on ageing at Stanford University

Expert Advice on How to Exercise

Often you may ask yourself, "why aren't you closing in on your ideal weight?" You're trying to workout and exercise, but your bathroom scale is not showing you any results – your weight appears the same as when you started out. Here are some tips from the fitness experts:

1. An effective weekly exercise program should get your heart pumping. Include one rigorous program that makes you sweat; two moderate exercise programs, and one easy session. For example: take an aerobics or Zumba workout class and then a more relaxing yoga class.

2. Drink at least 64 ounces (2 quarts) of distilled water daily. Drinking water has a huge effect on exercise. Dehydrated exercisers worked out 25% less effectively than those who drank water before and during workouts.

3. In the initial phases of exercise training, you may get post-workout dips in blood sugar that cause cravings for simple carbohydrates like sweets, etc. These cravings should disappear a few weeks into your exercise training. It's wise to have fresh fruit (apple, banana, orange, etc.) or trail mix available to prevent reaching for unhealthy sugar bars.

What Miracles Exercise Can Do For You

Get outdoors fast and get physically active when you feel dark moods, anxieties, worries, blues, depression and tensions overtaking you – otherwise these negative moods can damage you! Walking or any other outdoor exercise will help clear up your thinking and put your problems in perspective. Any form of outdoor recreation recreates the human personality. The ancient men of India who desired to become one with God believed the body and bloodstream had to be pure and strong before this could become a reality. Thus, they developed a physical fitness system called Yoga. They daily practice their belief that the body is meant to be stretched, strengthened and exercised correctly in order to remain healthy. No matter what your calendar years, start turning back your biological clock now faithfully with exercise.

Associate with health-minded friends who live a healthy lifestyle. Walk, talk and exercise together and enjoy similar healthy goals.

Benefits that Daily Exercise Can Bring You:

1. Exercise increases circulation, and brings more oxygen into your body. You will feel more energetic.

2. Exercise relieves stress, strain and tension. Tension gets locked in the tight, stiffened areas of your body, especially the neck, back and spine. Exercise will stretch and loosen these areas as it restores youthful limberness. You will feel more relaxed and at ease.

3. Overcoming chronic tiredness is a major benefit of exercise. That chronic tired feeling to a great extent is due to a lack of sufficient circulation to your brain. Exercise brings the oxygen-laden blood into this vital area with an energizing and revitalizing effect.

4. Exercise helps calm the nerves. Nothing can calm the nerves better than 30 minutes of brisk walking and exercise. It also helps to promote a good night's sleep, which is absolutely essential to maintaining calmness, repose, serenity, health and Nerve Force.

5. Exercise increases emotional control. Exercise helps to strengthen the nerves of the body and helps create the healthy composure that comes from a healthy nervous system and a balanced, happy state of mind.

Exercise Promotes Health & Youthfulness

We know that healthy living with proper exercise can produce a new breed of men and women who will enjoy more strength to carry out their daily work and have sufficient energy left for after-work interests, family and hobbies. They can retain the prime of life for 20 to 40 years longer than the person who is lazy and will not exercise! Examples: both Tom Selleck and Clint Eastwood have been proponents of exercise, lifting weights and eating healthy.

All external characteristics of health (such as powerful Nerve Force) are but the result of the healthy functioning of your vital internal organs and glands. These are what keep you going! Exercise actually reaches into your body bringing about miracle improvements in certain internal parts such as your nervous system, your heart, liver, lungs, kidneys, entire digestive tract, colon and thyroid gland among others. To attain these benefits you should faithfully follow a regular program of exercise.

Is age a hindrance to daily exercise? The answer is unequivocally, "No!" In fact, age is no excuse for not exercising! Our friend Roy White, 106 years young, walked 3 to 8 miles daily! (page 58). No one is too old to continue safe exercise!

To over rest is to rust! It's far better to wear out than to rust out. The saying, *If you don't use it, you lose it,* certainly applies to the body's 640 muscles. When you don't exercise regularly, your muscles lose their supple tone. As soon as you put down this book go outdoors and take a brisk, invigorating walk. Say out loud while walking: *Health! Peace! Joy! Love for Eternity!* You will feel great and your trillions of cells will rejoice with circulation!

Enjoy Exercising – It's Healthy and Fun!

There is great hiking near where we had a home in Hollywood, California, where Mt. Hollywood rises some 1,600 feet in famous Griffith Park. We enjoyed early morning hikes up the mountain to greet the sun rising and then would run down. Also, in Santa Barbara, CA, we always enjoyed an ocean swim and hiking in the surrounding foothills.

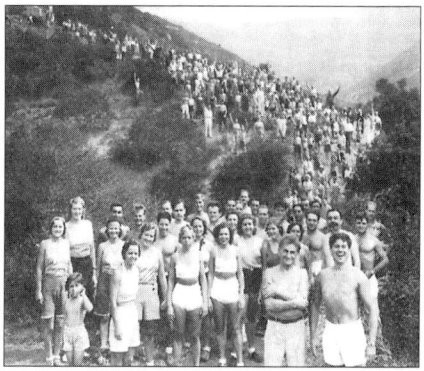

A thousand Happy Bragg Health Students enjoy hiking, exercise and fresh air on the trail to Mt. Hollywood, CA, summer, 1932.

We loved to walk, jog and climb mountains. We made time to walk or jog daily, or we swam, played tennis or rode our bikes. We worked out 3 times a week with a progressive weight training program, which helped keep our bones and muscles healthier and stronger. See pages 117 to 118.

Exercise is the greatest single health factor available to man that helps remove any blockages and unclog the arteries and blood vessels, and for increasing the vital flow of oxygen-enriched blood throughout the heart and body! Recent studies show that exercise improves health and also reduces the risk of developing adult-onset diabetes as well as breast cancer. The Harvard School of Public Health Researchers (*www.health.harvard.edu*) studied 70,000 women. Results: 46% lowered their risk of diabetes with daily vigorous exercising and brisk walking.

Enjoy Exercise and Jogs for Longer, Healthy Life

On our world Bragg Health Crusades the first question we would ask the hotel manager was, where is the nearest park where we can take our daily exercise? And off we would go sometime during the day. We preferred to go early in the morning or late in the afternoon. Each person, however, should choose the time best suited and available to them.

We are so pleased to find that all over the world today walking, hiking, running and jogging have become an accepted method in the pursuit of Heart Fitness by people of all age groups. Many cities have walking, hiking and jogging clubs. We have enjoyed running with folks world-wide; including Europe, England, Australia, New Zealand and throughout the USA.

It's universally accepted exercise is important for physical, mental and emotional health. A daily run or jog when adapted to an individual's physical condition and age will improve endurance, produce a sense of well-being and help to maintain total body fitness (each step gives your trillions of cells a massage). Also try trampolining and stationary jogging while watching TV. Exercise helps increase resistance to sickness and many diseases and helps make your body and heart stronger and life longer!

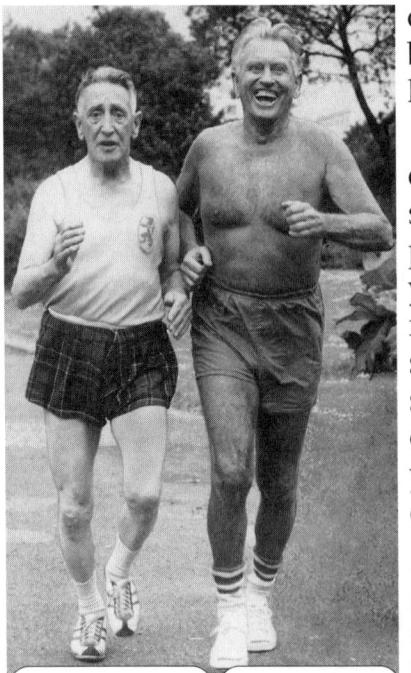

Duncan McLean | Paul C. Bragg

Before starting on your exercise program, it's wise to seek advice from your health practitioner. Also, be sure that you choose a soft surface to run or jog on, such as grass or sand. Jogging on hard surfaces, such as concrete and asphalt, could accumulate damage to your knees, hips, ankles and other organs.

Bragg with friend Duncan McLean, England's oldest Champion Sprinter, (83 years young) on a training run in London's beautiful Regent's Park.

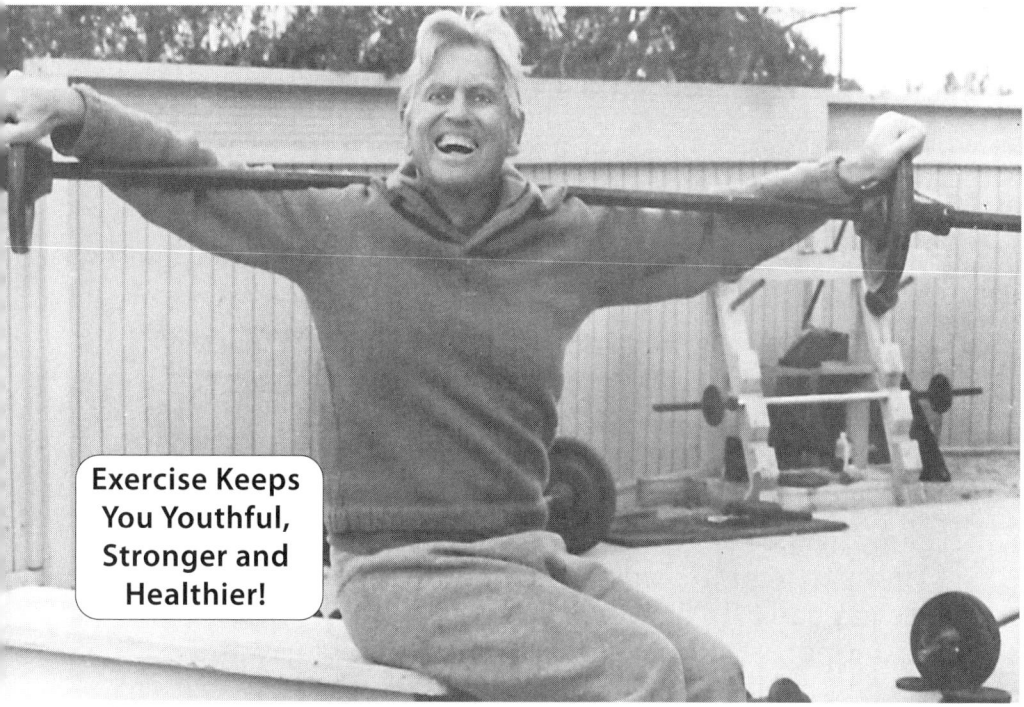

Paul C. Bragg and Patricia enjoyed lifting weights 3 times weekly.

Iron-Pumping Oldsters (ages 86 to 96) Triple Their Muscle Strength In Landmark U.S. Government Study

WASHINGTON NEWS — Ageing nursing home residents in Boston *pumping iron?* Elderly weightlifters tripling and quadrupling their muscle strength? Is it possible? Most people would doubt and wonder at this amazing revelation!

Yet the government experts on ageing answered those questions with a resounding *"yes"* according to the results of this study. They turned a group of frail Boston nursing home residents, aged 86 to 96, into weight-lifters to demonstrate that it's never too late to reverse age-related declines in muscle strength. The study group participated in a regime of high-intensity weight-training research conducted by the Agriculture Departments Human Research Center of Ageing at Tufts University in Boston. *A high-intensity weight training program is capable of inducing dramatic increases in the muscle strength in frail men and women up to 96 years of age.* This was reported by Dr. Maria A. Fiatarone, the Study Director.

The favorable response to strength training in these subjects was remarkable in light of their very advanced age, extremely sedentary habits, many chronic diseases, functional disabilities and nutritional inadequacies.

Despite their many handicaps, the elderly weight lifters increased their muscle strength by 3 to 4 times in as little as 8 weeks. Dr. Fiatarone said they were stronger at the end of the program than they had been in years!

Dr. Fiatarone and associates emphasized the safety of such a closely supervised weight lifting program, even among people in frail health. The average age of the ten participants was 90. Six had coronary heart disease, seven had arthritis, six had bone fractures resulting from osteoporosis, four had high blood pressure, and all had been physically inactive for years. Yet no serious medical problems resulted from this program. A few participants did report minor muscle and joint aches, but 9 of the 10 still completed the program.

The study participants, drawn from a 712-bed long-term care facility in Boston, worked out three times a week during the study. They performed three sets of eight repetitions with each leg on a weight lifting machine. The weights were gradually increased from 10 pounds to about 40 pounds at the end of the eight week program.

Dr. Fiatarone said the study carries potentially important implications for older people, who represent a growing proportion of the population. A decline in muscle strength and size is one of the more predictable features of ageing! Muscle strength in the average adult decreases by 30% to 50% during the course of a lifetime. Experts on ageing do not know whether the decrease is an unavoidable consequence of ageing, or results mainly from a sedentary lifestyle and other controllable factors.

Our friend, engineer Jim Cotton, back in 1969 started the "Waikiki Rough Water Swim Series" and dad enjoyed being in this event. Now there are close to 1,000 competitors yearly in this popular 2 mile rough water swim.

It's proven that exercise helps, but over 60% of U.S. adults do not get enough physical activity to help keep them healthy and fit.

More Muscles Linked to Longer Life

The more strong muscles older adults have, the lower their death risk, according to a new UCLA study. The findings add to growing evidence that overall body composition and not the widely used body mass index (BMI), is a better predictor of all-cause mortality. The greater your lean muscles, the lower risk of premature death; rather than worrying about weight or body mass index, people should be trying to maximize and maintain their lean muscle tissues. The studies show it appears to be an important predictor of risk of death. The researchers focused on a group of 3,659 individuals that included men who were 55 or older and women who were 65 or older. The study found that there needs to be focus on ways to improve body composition, rather than BMI alone, when counseling older adults on preventative health behaviors. Visit: *www.ScienceDaily.com*

The Benefits of Being Fit and Healthy

The benefits of being fit and keeping active, are an improved quality of life and being able to do things you enjoy for longer periods of time. To be fit, one must have good habits! This includes eating healthy foods like organic fruits and vegetables, exercising regularly, getting enough sleep and living clean! Becoming fit will help you tremendously both physically and mentally. As you become more fit these benefits will happen:

Looking Better: weight loss, toned muscles, better posture.

Feeling Better: more energy, better sleep, better able to cope with stress, reduced depression and anxiety, increased mental sharpness, fewer aches and pains.

Being Healthier: more efficient heart and lungs, lower cholesterol, lower blood pressure, ability to heal faster, stronger bones, less risk of osteoporosis, less stress on your joints, better balance and flexibility, strengthened immune system, reduced risk of dying early, diabetes, heart disease, obesity, cancers, stroke (*www.icb2001.com*).

Exercise, along with healthy foods and some fasting helps maintain or restore a healthy physical balance and normal weight for a long, happy life.

Exercise is the Best Fitness Conditioner

A daily program of walking, running or jogging is a quick, sure and inexpensive fitness conditioner. Be faithful to your exercise routine for true heart fitness. Women will be especially pleased when they see fat change to lean, as the inches fly off their waistlines and hip-lines – all the while improving their health! Men and women both, **please remember your waistline is your lifeline and also your dateline! A person with a trim and fit figure always looks more youthful and attractive!**

If you feel you cannot get outside for your run or jog on cold and rainy days – stationary inside jogging to music or your favorite show will work too. Stay in one place and lift one foot at a time about 6-8 inches from floor – it's best to start easy and gradually build up to faster, longer periods. Remember to exercise where you get the most fresh air – on the patio, front porch, or inside or outside rest areas at work.

The Miracle Life of Ageless Jack LaLanne

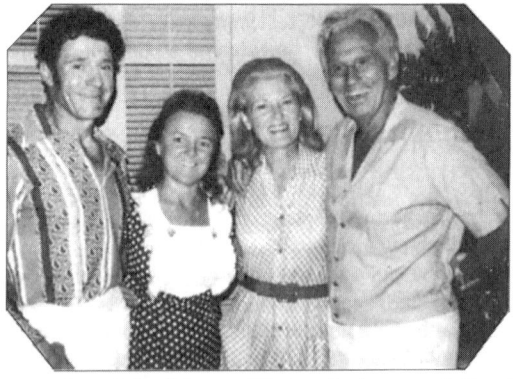

Jack LaLanne, Patricia Bragg, Elaine LaLanne & Paul C. Bragg

Jack says he would have been dead by 16 if he hadn't attended the Bragg Crusade. Jack says, *"Bragg saved my life at age 15, when I attended the Bragg Health and Fitness Crusade in Oakland, California."* From that day on, Jack continued to live The Bragg Healthy Lifestyle, and inspired millions to health, fitness and a long fulfilled, happy life! Visit *JackLalanne.com.*

For an instant mood lifter, take a brisk walk counting your blessings. Exercise and fresh air have positive effects on the human spirit and mind.

Macfadden – Founder of Physical Culture

My dad worked closely with Bernarr Macfadden and together they changed the entire health culture in America. While Dad was the father of the Health Movement and the originator of health food stores, Macfadden was known as the father of physical culture in America. He founded the *"Physical Culture Magazine,"* the first of its kind in the country. My father served as the editor of the magazine, which brought the basic principles of healthful living to popular attention in America. They were credited with "getting women out of bloomers into shorts, and men into bathing trunks." Macfadden started "Penny Kitchen Restaurants" during the big Depression Era, when they fed millions of hungry people for a penny each. Bragg helped Macfadden with his Miami Health Spa Hotel: The Macfadden – Deauville Hotel.

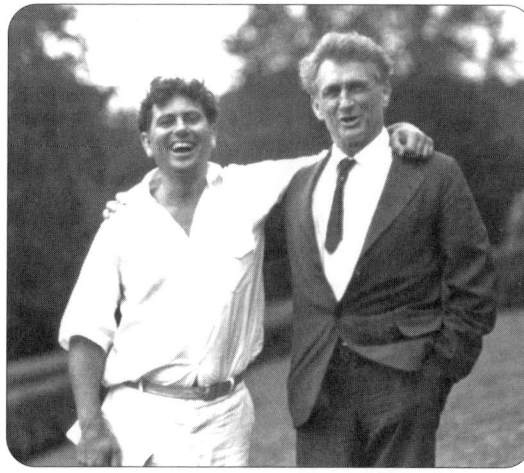

Paul Bragg & Mentor – Bernarr Macfadden

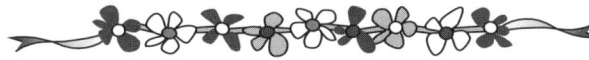

Here's Dad with Bernarr Macfadden, who spent thousands of dollars to find the *oldest living humans* on earth. Dad was his main researcher. This took him to many interesting, remote parts of the world, interviewing men and women from *100 to 120 years of age!* Dad found this work fascinating, because he loved promoting health and longevity – an active life that could last 120 to 150 years (Genesis 6:3). The Bragg research proved it can be done! Now Scientists worldwide are agreeing.

Healthy Heart Habits for Long, Vital Life

Remember, *organic live foods make live people. You are what you eat, drink, breathe, think, say and do.* **So eat a low-fat, low-sugar, high-fiber diet of organic fresh raw salads, sprouts, greens, vegetables, whole grains, fruits, raw seeds, nuts, fresh juices and chemical-free, purified or distilled water.**

Earn your food with daily exercise. For regular exercise, brisk walking, improves your health, stamina, go-power, flexibility, endurance and helps open the cardiovascular system! Only 45 minutes a day truly can do miracles for your heart, arteries, mind, nerves, soul and body! You become revitalized with new zest for living to accomplish your life goals!

We are made of tubes. To help keep them open, clean and to maintain good elimination, I take 1 veg psyllium cap or add 1 tsp psyllium husk powder daily an hour after dinner to juices, herbal teas, even apple cider vinegar drink. I also take one Cayenne capsule (40,000 HU) daily with a meal. I take 50 to 100 mgs. regular-released Niacin (B3) with one meal daily to help cleanse and open the cardiovascular system; also improves memory. Skin flushing may occur, don't worry about this as it shows it's working! After cholesterol level reaches 180, then only take Niacin twice weekly.

The heart needs healthy balanced nutrients, so take natural multi-vitamin-mineral food supplements: Omega-3 and extra heart helpers – vitamin E with mixed tocotrienols; vitamin C; Ubiquinol CoQ10; vitamin D3; MSM; D-Ribose; garlic; turmeric; selenium; zinc; beta carotene and amino acids – L-Carnitine, L-Taurine, L-Lysine and Proline. Folic acid, CoQ10, vitamin B6 and B12 helps keep homocysteine level low. Magnesium orotate, hawthorn berry extract helps bring relief for palpitations, arrhythmia, senile hearts and coronary disease. Take multi-digestive enzyme and probiotics with meals; it aids in digestion, assimilation and elimination.

For sleep problems try 5-HTP tryptophan (an amino acid), melatonin, calcium, magnesium, valerian (in capsule, extract or tea), and Sleepytime herb tea. For arthritis or joint pain/stiffness, try aloe juice or gel, glucosamine-chondroitin-MSM combo caps and shots, helps heal and regenerate. Capsaicin and DMSO lotion helps relieve pain. Natural liver cleanses to repair and regenerate include: milk thistle; dandelion root; artichoke and turmeric. Dandelion root is a natural diuretic and helps clear toxins through urination and also helps stimulate liver bile flow so waste can be eliminated.

Use amazing antioxidants – E Tocotrienols, vitamin C, quercetin, grape seed extract (OPCs), CoQ10, selenium, SOD, resveratrol, and alpha-lipoic acid. They improve immune system and help flush out dangerous free radicals that cause havoc with cardiovascular pipes and health. Research shows antioxidants promote longevity, slow ageing, fight toxins, help prevent disease, cancer, cataracts and exhaustion.

Recommended Heart Health Tests (for Adults):

- **Total Cholesterol:** 180 mg/dl or less is optimal
- **LDL Cholesterol:** 130 mg/dl or less is optimal • **HDL Cholesterol:** 50 mg/dl or more
- **Triglycerides:** 150 mg/dl or less is normal level
- **HDL/Cholesterol Ratio:** 5.0 or less • **Triglycerides/HDL Ratio:** below 2
- **Homocysteine:** 6-9 micromoles/L
- **CRP** (**C-Reactive Protein high sensitivity**):
  - 1 mg/L = low risk • 1-3 mg/L = average risk • over 3 mg/L = high risk
- **Diabetic Risk Tests:**
  - **Glucose:** (do 12 hour food fast) 80-100 mg/dl • **Hemoglobin A1c:** 6% or less
- **Blood Pressure:** 120/70 mmHg is good for adults

Correct Breathing

Fifth Step Towards Powerful Nerve Force

Oxygen-starved people are usually nervous people with many problems. As we have discussed, the activity of the vital organs depends directly upon the nerve stimulus they receive from the nervous system. Nerve Exhaustion therefore impairs the action of the stomach, kidneys, bowels and other abdominal organs, causing digestive distress and other innumerable body ailments.

The heart and lungs are especially affected by Nerve Exhaustion and tension! We all have observed that the slightest excitement will speed up heart beat, blood pressure and breathing. Fear and worry depress the action of the heart and lungs, an effect which can become quite serious! The heart and lungs – upon which life depends more directly than any other organs – may be considered the master organs of the miracle body! When the heart stops beating, death will result in a few minutes, and the heart will stop beating soon after its oxygen supply is shut off.

The blood is your river of life and it must be kept pure! It's one of the main duties of the heart and lungs to do this important task. With each breath, life-giving oxygen is carried into the blood, while carbon dioxide is transported away.

When You Breathe Deeply and Fully You Live Longer and Healthier

Air is the body's most important energizer. The more deeply you breathe pure air, the better your chances are for extending your life. For over 85 years, we have done extensive research on long-lived people and we've discovered this common denominator: they are all deep breathers. We have found that the deeper, fewer breaths a person takes in one minute, the longer they live. Most rapid breathers are short-lived. **It's essential and life-enhancing that we breathe deeply and correctly for super health.**

The Lower Respiratory System

Your Lungs Are Miracles – Be Good To Them!

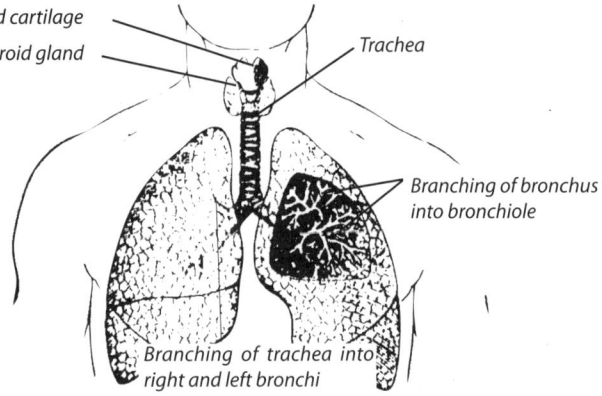

Path of Breath

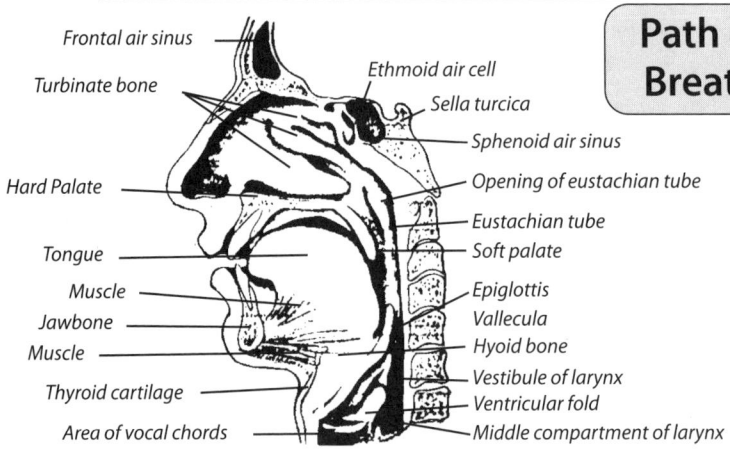

Mechanics of Breathing

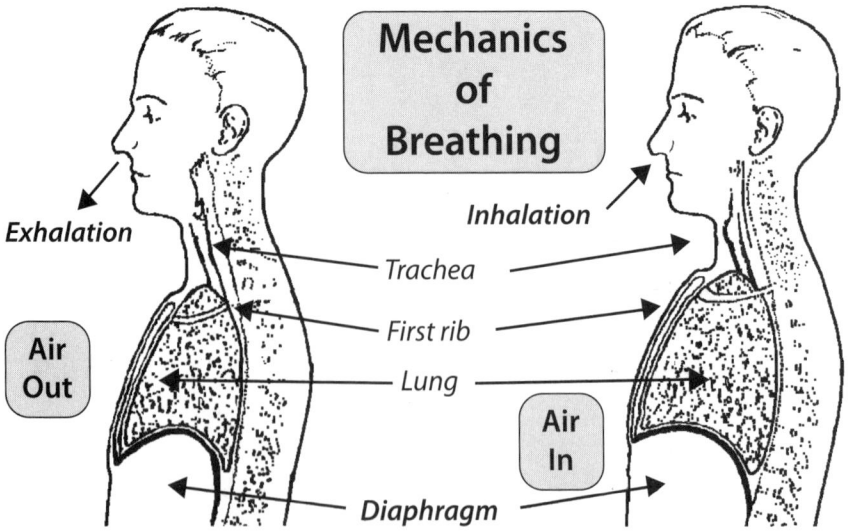

Mechanics of Breathing, showing Diaphragm Position and Flexible Ribs at Out Exhalation and at Inhalation.

Shallow Breathers Self-Poison Themselves

When you are a shallow breather, you don't change the air at the base of your lungs, where two-thirds of your lung capacity is located. When you return impure blood to your body, the ill effects are compounded because your blood cannot perform properly. It's difficult for blood that's loaded with poisonous wastes to transport the relatively small amount of oxygen which it absorbs; it's even harder for it to carry necessary nourishment from food. **An inadequate oxygen supply impairs your body's ability to break down food into digestible elements. This slows all bodily function! This is why deep breathing is vitally important for health!**

With the wrong diet and shallow breathing, the organs of elimination are overworked and underfed! But accumulating wastes must go somewhere. Some are discharged into sweat glands. This toxic overload produces unpleasant body odors! Other toxic wastes end up deposited as heavy mucus into sinus cavities, lungs and bronchial tubes. Some line the passages of the ears, eyes, nose and throat, as well as along the digestive tract. Deposits of hardened wastes in moveable joints can cause pressure on nerves, creating painful warning signals. **Pain is Mother Nature's flashing red warning signal that something is wrong in your body!** This pain warning should be respected with corrective measures taken right away – not repressed by painkilling drugs full of both known and unknown side-effects!

Shallow breathers actually poison themselves by robbing their bodies of sufficient oxygen! This is auto-intoxication (self-poisoning). They are slowly suffocating and dying in their own body wastes and poisons. **Pneumonia is a shocking example; body and lungs fill up and drown in their own toxins and mucus.**

Consider this: if someone tried to force you to kill yourself by taking shallow breaths, what would you do? You'd fight back! In defiance, you would breathe deeply, cleansing your blood and entire miracle body system to give your body more life, energy and super health!

Breathing is the greatest pleasure in life! – Papini, 1881-1956

What is Diaphragmatic Breathing?

Diaphragmatic Breathing – sometimes called "abdominal breathing" is entirely different in action from chest breathing. During inhalation the abdomen expands (becomes larger) and during exhalation the abdomen contracts (becomes smaller). It must be understood that air does not enter the abdominal region with this form of breathing. This is impossible.

How to Practice Diaphragmatic Breathing

It's best to begin practicing Diaphragmatic Breathing while lying down since it's more easily performed in this position. After faithfully practicing for a few weeks lying down, then do your regular practice while you are sitting or standing. **Continue your conscious Diaphragmatic Breathing until full control is attained naturally over the diaphragm and it becomes a healthy unconscious habit!** Conscious Diaphragmatic Breathing is of great help in restoring the heart action to normal. Heart fluttering, skipping of beats and other abnormal manifestations in heart action are very common in people with damaged nerves. We know of many cases in which Diaphragmatic Breathing helped correct the most serious forms of so-called "heart trouble." The habit of Diaphragmatic Breathing should be acquired as quickly as possible because it is a primary requisite for Supreme Health, whether or not one is the victim of "negative stress."

Advantages of Diaphragmatic Breathing:

1. **Helps to detoxify the body.** Relieves pain. Increases cardiovascular capacity. Stimulates the lymphatic system. Promotes greater oxygenation of the blood.

2. **Makes you calmer and happier.** Gives you energy. Improves your digestion. Helps improve your posture. Strengthens your major organs. Helps regulate your weight. Lowers your chances of sickness and disease.

Your brain, which requires 3 times more oxygen than the rest of your body, suffers first. 55% of delinquent behavior in minors can be attributed to oxygen starvation. – Dr. Philip Rice, specialist with delinquent children

3. Stimulation of Peristalsis – the worm-like motion of the intestines – which promotes digestion and then the elimination of toxic fecal wastes. We know of hundreds of cases in which a change from chest to Diaphragmatic Breathing helped to correct long standing conditions including chronic constipation, gas, heartburn, indigestion and liver troubles.

4. A remarkably healthy calming effect upon the nerves – especially pneumogastric nerve and solar plexus. Diaphragmatic Breathing breaks up the paralyzing nerve tension so often observed in people with super-sensitive or damaged nerves. The close relation between the pneumogastric nerve, breathing and the vital organs is demonstrated when a baby is born. In an unborn child in the womb, the vital organs are practically at a standstill. If food were in the stomach, it would not be digested, but with the first breath – the "Breath of Life" – the baby's entire vital machinery is then set in motion! This breath means the awakening of the pneumogastric nerve and especially the solar plexus.

Control Jagged, Jumpy Nerves With Long, Slow Diaphragmatic Breathing

Many things can trigger the nerves into a heightened emotional state – worries and cares of all kinds, grief, emotional shock, stress, strain and tension. Family relationships can bring on nervous upsets. Husbands and wives who can't communicate have great emotional battles. Parents and children often find the generation gap so wide they can't bridge it and this produces frustrations. Marital or in-law problems, financial worries and sickness can all trigger an emotional upset and stress.

Here's how to restore balance to the nervous system when an emotional upset strikes you. Go to a quiet place, even if you have to go into a closet. First just sit still. Take your pulse rate. You will find it's racing. You will also find during emotional excitement you will take rapid chest breaths.

During stress or anger, we tend to inhale and hold our breath. The therapeutic aspect of this breathing is exhalation – which is at least twice the length of inhalation. The exhalation alerts the body it can relax and resume essential peaceful body functions.

Long, Slow Diaphragmatic Breathing Leads to a Long, Peaceful, Healthy Life!

Miracles happen when you slow down your breathing. Take full diaphragmatic breaths. See how few long, slow deep breaths you can take in a minute. After a few minutes you will find your pulse rate is slower. Your nerves begin to quiet down. Instead of trying to solve your emotional problems in a state of excitement, you are now calm! This long, slow Diaphragmatic Breathing allows you to shift from emotionalism to logical thinking. You become master of the situation. You no longer look at your problems subjectively, but begin to take the broad, objective view. With logical and positive thinking you can find the answers to emotional problems. If you use this technique when emotional shocks hit, you'll save yourself a lot of lost Nerve Force. This slow, deep Diaphragmatic Breathing is a wonderful method to calm yourself and weather life's emotional upsets.

The shortest lived animals are those who breathe rapidly. The longest lived animals are those who take slower breaths. Many years ago we learned this secret from a Breatharian – as he was known – who lived in India. It was claimed by many that he was over 130 years of age! He looked like a well preserved man in his early 70s. He had sharp eyes and a wrinkle-free face with a happy disposition and a keen mind. He could tell you what had happened in his life 125 years ago!

He practiced long, slow Diaphragmatic Breathing and did it so well that he took only one full breath per minute. He was an Indian Guru, a teacher and had attained perfect bliss consciousness. He finally went to a retreat in the Himalayan Mountains. Dad and I are students of deep breathing and we practiced it daily. We are aware of how important oxygen (the invisible staff of life) is to our well-being and to the building of our bodies' powerful Nerve Force and super health.

TEST See if you are a Chest Breather? OR Abdomen Breather? Place right hand on chest and left hand on abdomen. As you breathe, see which hand rises more. If right hand rises more, you are a chest breather. If left hand rises more, you are an abdomen breather.

Deadly Smoking – Health Hazard to Avoid – What it Does to You & Those Around You!

When people inhale deadly tobacco smoke into their miracle lungs, the protective cilia hairs filter out much of the smoke's harmful substances before it is exhaled. This means that while harmful toxins are trapped in the delicate linings of the smokers' lungs, fewer of these toxins are re-released into the air for others to breathe in. However, between a smoker's deadly puffs, the cigarette burns directly into the air. This smoke is known as "secondhand, side-stream" smoke, but it should be called "direct" smoke. Smoke that burns directly into the air is completely unfiltered and more deadly than the smokers' smoke! **Stay away from all deadly smoke!**

Recent studies establish that people who live or work around smokers are more likely to develop lung, asthma and sinus damage than smokers. For asthma or bronchitis sufferers, this exposure is very damaging! In addition to these dangers, "direct" smoke irritates the eyes, nose and throat and smells up everything it touches (rooms, hotels, offices, carpets, drapes, cars and everything around smoking).

For the cigarette smoker, whose miracle lungs have unfortunately become the filters protecting the body from the deadly smoke, the effects are equally – if not more – damaging! Tar begins to collect in the lungs once there is too much to be removed through the lungs' normal cleaning processes. This means the over-burdened lungs can no longer clean normal contaminants they have to deal with. Dirt inhaled into the alveoli – which is normally trapped in a layer of sticky mucus and carried out of the lungs by the wavelike motions of the tiny cilia hairs – becomes trapped and stuck in the lungs. The cilia hairs become paralyzed by tar, so the normal cleansing (drain) procedures break down and the airways become clogged. This makes the lungs resort to coughing, spitting and respiratory-breathing attacks, flu, etc. in an effort to expel the contaminated, clogging toxins, tar and mucus.

There is good news. When a person stops smoking the cilia hairs begin to heal and move again. Smokers – stop now, you begin cleansing and healing immediately!

DEADLY SMOKING FACTS – Reasons to Stop!

- Tobacco use and also second-hand smoke will eventually kill over one fifth of the world population – now 6 million yearly.
- Of the over 50 million Americans who smoke, one third to one half will die from a smoke-related disease and all will reduce their life expectancy by an average of nine years.
- Smoking acts as either a stimulant or a depressant – depending upon the smoker's emotional state at the time.
- The average pack-a-day smoker takes about 92,000 *hits* of deadly nicotine each year. Do visit and read: *www.ash.org*
- "Second hand smoke" hurts non-smokers: it speeds up their heart rate, raises blood pressure and doubles the amount of deadly carbon monoxide in their blood. It's a killer!
- Secondary deadly smoke contains more nicotine, tar and cadmium than mainstream smoke (leads to hypertension, emphysema, cancer, and asthma) and is killing millions!
- Babies born to mothers who smoke tend to have lower body weight, smaller lungs, poor health and many develop asthma.
- Lung illnesses are twice as common in smokers' children.
- Children and teenagers make up 90% of the new smokers in the United States – and teenage (deadly) smoking is on the rise!
- The death rate from breast cancer ranges from 25% to 75% higher among women who smoke. *www.BreastCancer.org*
- Female smokers may face a higher risk of lung cancer – as much as twice the risk of male smokers, according to a study done by Dr. Harvey Risch at Yale University.
- For both men and women, those who smoked more than two packs a day were 50 times more likely to develop lung cancer than those who never smoked (*National Cancer Institute*).
- Your body contains almost 100,000 miles of blood vessels. Smoking ages and constricts those vessels, depriving your body of important, rich oxygen it needs, lack causes serious illness.
- Tobacco is the main introduction to more deadly drugs!!!
- Teens who smoke are far more likely to engage in other risky and life-threatening behaviors than non-smoking healthy teens.
- Cataracts, cancer, angina, arteriosclerosis, osteoporosis, chronic bronchitis, asthma, high blood pressure, impotency and respiratory ailments are linked to all forms of smoking.

QUIT SMOKING! All smokers must stop this vicious, deadly smoking habit that destroys health, youth, energy and life!

Quit Smoking – See the Difference it Makes!

- **20 MINUTES AFTER QUITTING:** Your blood pressure, heart rate and pulse rate drop to normal levels. The temperature of your hands and feet increases to normal.
- **8 HOURS AFTER QUITTING:** Carbon monoxide (which can be toxic to your body) decreases to lower levels and your blood oxygen levels increase to normal.
- **24 HOURS AFTER QUITTING:** You substantially lessen your chances of having a heart attack or stroke.
- **48 HOURS AFTER QUITTING:** Your nerve endings start regrowing and your ability to taste and smell is enhanced.
- **2 WEEKS TO 3 MONTHS AFTER QUITTING:** Nicotine will now be out of your body. Your circulation improves. Brisk walking, physical activity and exercise becomes easier. Your lung function increases as much as 30%.
- **1 TO 9 MONTHS AFTER QUITTING:** You will be able to exercise and perform physical activities without feeling winded and sick. Coughing, sinus congestion, fatigue and shortness of breath decreases. Your lungs and body are becoming cleaner and more resistant to infection.
- **1 YEAR AFTER QUITTING:** You will no longer have withdrawal symptoms. Excess risk for coronary heart disease decreases to an amazing 50% that of a smoker's.
- **2 TO 3 YEARS AFTER QUITTING:** Risk for heart disease and stroke decrease compared to those of people who have never smoked. Also less chance of osteoporosis.
- **5 YEARS AFTER QUITTING:** Lung cancer death rate for former one-pack-a-day smoker decreases by almost half. Risk of having a stroke reduces, risk of developing mouth and throat cancer is half that of a smoker.
- **10 TO 15 YEARS AFTER QUITTING:** Lung cancer death rate is almost that of non-smokers. Pre-cancerous cells are replaced. Risks for mouth, throat, esophagus, bladder, kidney, breast and pancreas cancer have decreased. Risk of developing diabetes is now similar to that of a person who has never smoked.

– Prevention Magazine • www.prevention.com

Heimlich Maneuver Jumpstarts the Lungs

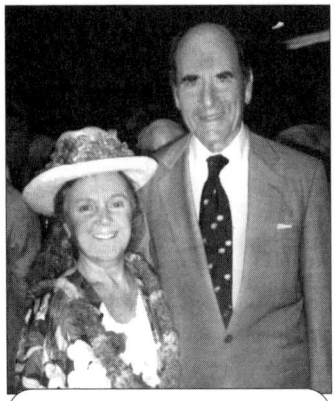

Dr. Henry Heimlich & Patricia Bragg in Honolulu

My father and I want to do all we can to ensure that all people are able to get the oxygen they need.

Many of you are familiar with the famous Heimlich Maneuver as a technique for saving choking victims. Since 1974, this procedure has saved over 100,000 lives just in the United States. This maneuver, developed by Dr. Henry Heimlich, is performed by pressing upward on the diaphragm. This compresses the lungs, causing a flow of air that helps push the choking object out that is blocking the airway. Recent evidence and research has suggested the Heimlich Maneuver is effective in restoring breathing in more emergency situations than just choking. Our friends Dr. Heimlich along with his wife Jane Murray Heimlich *(the daughter of famous Arthur and Katherine Murray who taught America to dance)* dedicated their lives to educating the world about the life-saving Heimlich Maneuver.

Heimlich Helps Save Drowning Victims

In more than 90% of drowning cases, the victim's lungs fill with fluid. In this situation, it's imperative that the fluid be expelled quickly - because after four or five minutes the likelihood of brain damage increases. Just getting someone out of the water has not changed their condition – if they still have fluid in their lungs their condition is the same as if they were still under water. In all the studies on drowning since 1933, none showed that mouth-to-mouth resuscitation saved drowning victims without first draining water from their lungs. After all, air cannot get into water-filled lungs!

The Heimlich Maneuver expels water from lungs of drowning victims in six to nine seconds – with two to four Heimlich applications. And unlike CPR, when applied correctly, Heimlich is safe and easily mastered by a person new to the procedure.

Bathing & Circulation

Sixth Step Towards Powerful Nerve Force

To build powerful Nerve Force we must be clean not only on the inside of our bodies, but on the outside as well. The Bragg Healthy Lifestyle recognizes that a program of eating live, clean and organic foods combined with deep breathing exercises and a fasting program, are all necessary for keeping our bodies healthy, clean and free from toxic poisons.

The body is constantly eliminating toxic poisons through skin pores. **Skin is the largest organ of the human body and one of the most important organs of elimination (often called the third kidney). Your skin has 96 million pores and they must be kept clean to function properly.** Bathing is important not only for cleansing the pores, but is also as an aid in building greater Nerve Force.

The toxic poisons come out through the pores of the skin in the form of moisture or water which dries on the skin. This residue must be washed away. That is why it's important to take daily cleansing baths or showers.

We personally think a shower is the best way to cleanse the skin. A shower head that has satisfactory pressure – can vary from a fine spray to a forceful spray of water – and also has an important filter is the best option.

Your choice of soap is also important. We don't use ordinary commercial soaps, but only pure Castile or veggie and herb soaps with an acid base. You see, it's important not to use alkaline soaps on the body because a healthy skin has an acid base. If you use ordinary soap which is alkaline, you wash away the healthful acid base of the skin. Your skin then gets dry and often becomes irritated, and a lot of Nerve Force is lost this way.

You can save yourself much money and the anxiety of falling ill by paying attention to your body's constant need for pure water.
– Dr. F. Batmanghelidj, author "Your Body's Many Cries For Water"

Cold Water on the Skin is Important For Building Powerful Nerve Force

Cold water – like pure, clean air – is a natural stimulant with no side effects if the body is conditioned to take cold water. After you have washed your body, then you can gradually make the shower colder and colder. After you get conditioned to a cold bath, you will revel in it! Cold water has a great strengthening effect on the nerves.

Also – for even better Nerve Force building – use a coarse dry washcloth to dry yourself at the end of your shower like a hand massage. Using this on the body while it is wet is a great nerve builder. After your body is almost dried finish with a large coarse bath towel and give your body another healthy thorough rubbing massage with it.

Cold water, hand rub drying, towel rubbing and skin brushing are all tonics to the nerves in the skin. You will tingle with vitality after you make this a part of your daily Bragg Healthy Lifestyle and Exercise Program!

Special Shower Builds Healthy Circulation

Here's a progressive method for improving circulation over your entire body. All you need is a large back brush or Swedish bath friction mitt, Castile soap and a coarse Turkish towel. Now get into the shower and turn on hot water. With brush or mitt, gently scrub your body. At first your coddled body won't be able to take too much scrubbing. It's also good to hand massage your neck and upper shoulders. After scrub/massage, then start to alternate hot and cold showers for 3 to 5 minutes. Now rub dry your body for 3 to 5 minutes – your body circulation will tingle!

Hot/cold water showers are a wonderful way to relax, refresh and stimulate tired muscles. Let the spray beat heavily on your back and shoulders. Occasionally before showering apply olive oil if your skin is dry. We advise this relaxing shower before dinner on days when you come home tired. It helps relieve muscular stress and strain!

We can no more afford to spend major time on minor things, than we can to spend minor time on major things!
– Jim Rohn, American entrepreneur, author and motivational speaker.

Cold Water Swimmers Are Fit and Ageless

My father prided himself on being able to endure the coldest weather wearing only a small amount of clothing, and he enjoyed swimming in all parts of the world, in all kinds of weather, (which I have also enjoyed). He was well known for his cold water swimming and was welcomed as a member at *Polar Bear Clubs* worldwide. On many occasions, Dad and famous pioneer Dr. Robert Jackson had great sport breaking the ice and swimming with the amazing *Boston Brownies* of the famous "L" Street Bath House in Massachusetts. Here you'd find some of the finest ageless physical specimens in the world, including people in their 60's, 70's, 80's 90's, and even over 100 years.

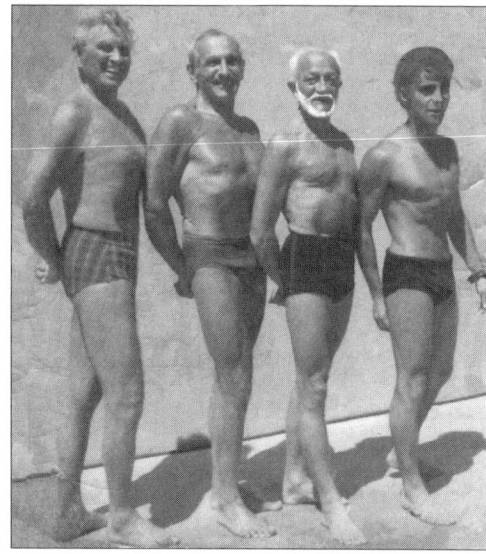

Cold Water Swimmers "L" Street Beach, Boston
Dr. Paul C. Bragg and Dr. John H. Federkiewicz,
David Cooper and Dr. David Carmos (the youngest)

The same is true of the *Polar Bear*s of Coney Island and at Montrose Beach in Chicago and those at the popular Bradford Beach in Milwaukee, Wisconsin. They were fit, amazing and ageless swimmers. We observed that many of those people who bathed all winter long in the icy waters of the Atlantic Ocean developed the most beautiful skin tone. It really was "the skin you love to touch." One winter Dad and I arrived in New York during a blizzard and found the members of the *Polar Bears* and *Iceberg Club* of Coney Island (both year round bathing clubs) out in full force and we joined them! These robust bathers displayed incredible Vital Nerve Force and had marvelous skin tone.

Now, we're not advising you to join a year round bather's club, but we are telling you that when the body is conditioned to cold water, there is stronger Nerve Force. That is the reason we want you to condition your body to cold water. It's a great tonic and a natural stimulant.

Warm and Hot Baths also Have Their Place in Building Nerve Force

There is a time for cold water bathing and a time for warm or hot bathing. When a person has a strenuous day and a great deal of Nerve Force has been expended and their nerves are keyed up and if their entire nervous system has been subjected to stress, strain and tension and their nerves feel as if they were tied in knots . . . this is not the time for a cold water bath! This is definitely a time to take a hot bath – around 102° to 104°F. There is nothing quite as soothing as when you snuggle down into a tub of warm water (add 1 cup vinegar) and let your whole body and nervous system unwind and relax.

We are devotees of both the cold and hot water bath. We had a home in Desert Hot Springs near Palm Springs where mineral water comes out of ground as hot as 167°F. Naturally, you can't bathe in this intense heat, but at the spas we have frequented, hot water is cooled to 104°F. We found it wonderful for our nerves to bathe in this hot mineral water. These health spas also have special soaking pools to enjoy and have swimming pools in which the mineral water is kept at 90°F. In this water, swimming is a real tonic for your entire nervous system.

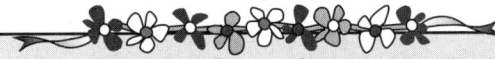

Prayer for Strength and Loving Guidance

I give thanks each day to live a simple, sincere and serene life; repelling promptly every thought of impurity, discontent, anxiety, discouragement and fear. I will continually cultivate health, cheerfulness, happiness, charity and the love of brotherhood; exercising economy in expenditure, generosity in giving, carefulness in conversation and diligence in appointed service. I pledge fidelity to every trust and a childlike faith in God while, in particular, I will be faithful in those habits of prayer, study, work, nutrition, physical exercise, deep breathing and good posture. I shall fast for 24 hours each week, eat only natural foods and get sufficient recharging sleep nightly. I will make every effort to improve myself physically, mentally, emotionally and spiritually every day.

– Prayer used by Paul C. Bragg and daughter Patricia Bragg

"Water contains healing; it is the simplest, cheapest and – if used correctly – the safest remedy. Water is my best friend and will remain all my life!"
– Father Sebastian Kneipp, Father of Hydrotherapy • www.Kneipp.com

Five Hidden Dangers in Your Shower:

• **Chlorine:** Added to all municipal water supplies, this disinfectant hardens arteries, destroys proteins in the body, irritates skin and sinus conditions and aggravates any asthma, allergies and respiratory problems.

• **Chloroform:** This powerful by-product of chlorination causes excessive free radical formation (a cause of accelerated ageing!) It causes normal cells to mutate and cholesterol to form. It's a known carcinogen!

• **DCA (Dichloroacetic acid):** This chlorine by-product alters cholesterol metabolism and has been shown to cause liver cancer in lab animals.

• **MX (a chlorinated acid)**: Another by-product of chlorination, MX is known to cause genetic mutations that can lead to cancer growth and has been found in all chlorinated water for which it was tested.

• **Proven cause of bladder and rectal cancer:** Research proved that chlorinated water is the direct cause of 9% of all U.S. bladder cancers and 15% of all rectal cancers.

Use Shower Filter to Remove Toxins

The most effective method of removing hazards from your shower is the quick and easy installation of a filter on your shower arm. The best filter we have found removes chlorine, lead, mercury, iron, chlorine by-products, arsenic, hydrogen sulfide, and many other unseen contaminants, such as bacteria, fungi, dirt and toxic sediments. It should have a 12 to 18 month life-span and be easily cleaned by backwashing and replaced when needed. I have been using this type of filter for many years and really enjoy my chlorine-free showers!

Start enjoying safe, chlorine-free showers right away. It's essential to reducing your risk of heart disease and cancer and to ease the strain on your immune system. You may even get rid of long-standing conditions – from sinus and respiratory problems, to dry, itchy skin.

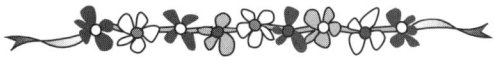

We grow healthier in life with safe pure water, healthy foods and love!

Prevention is always preferable to the cure.

Showers, Toxic Chemicals and Chlorine

Water chlorination has been widely used to "purify" water in America starting in 1904. But chlorine's negative effects on health surely outweigh any benefits! *"Chlorine is the greatest crippler and killer of modern times! While it prevented epidemics of one disease, it was creating another. Twenty years after the start of chlorinating our drinking water, the present mounting epidemic of heart trouble, cancer and senility began in 1924, and is costing billions."*
– Dr. Joseph Price, *Coronaries, Cholesterol, Chlorine*

Skin absorption of toxic dangerous contaminants has been greatly underestimated and the ingestion may not constitute the sole primary route of toxic exposure.
– Dr. Halina Brown, *American Journal of Public Health, 1984*

Taking long hot showers is a health risk, according to the latest research. Showers – and to a lesser extent baths – lead to a greater exposure to toxic chemicals contained in water supplies than does drinking the water. These toxic chemicals evaporate out of the water and are inhaled. They can also spread through the house and be inhaled by others. People get six to 100 times more chemicals by breathing the air while taking showers and baths than they would by drinking the water.
– Ian Anderson, *New Scientist*

A Professor of Water Chemistry at the University of Pittsburgh claims that exposure to vaporized chemicals in the water through showering, bathing and inhalation is 100 times greater than through drinking the chemicals in water.
– The Nader Report – Troubled Waters on Tap

CHECK FOLLOWING WEBSITES FOR FLUORIDE UPDATES:

- **www.FluorideAlert.org** • **fluoride.mercola.com**
- **www.slweb.org/bibliography.html**
- **www.DoctorYourself.com/carton.html**

THE LAW OF CAUSE AND EFFECT: An unhealthy lifestyle produces illnesses and disease. Most humans are lacking good nutrition and pure water to maintain optimum health! Fact: most people are dehydrated. Eight glasses of distilled water daily is vital to operate body functions, brain, nerves, energy, etc. and to achieve Powerful Nerve Force for Super Health! – Paul C. Bragg, N.D., Ph.D., Life Extension Specialist & Originator Health Stores

You Get More Toxic Exposure from Taking a Chlorinated Water Shower Than From Drinking the Same Water!

Two of the very highly toxic and volatile chemicals, trichloroethylene and chloroform, have been proven as toxic contaminants found in most all municipal drinking U.S. water supplies. The National Academy of Sciences has estimated that hundreds of people die in the United States each year from the cancers caused largely by ingesting water pollutants from inhalation as air pollutants in the home. Inhalation exposure to water pollutants is largely ignored. Recent shocking data indicates that hot showers can liberate about 50% of the chloroform and 80% of the trichloroethylene into the air.

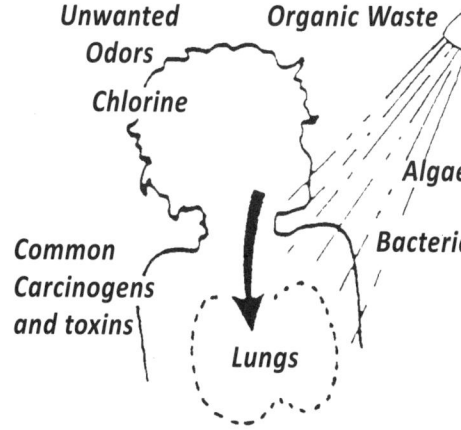

Tests show your body can absorb more toxic chlorine from a 10 minute shower than drinking 8 glasses of the same water. How can that be? A warm shower opens up your pores, causing your skin to act like a sponge. As a result, you not only inhale the toxic chlorine vapors, you absorb them through your skin, directly into your bloodstream – at a toxic rate that is up to 6 times higher than drinking it.

In terms of cumulative damage to your health, showering in chlorinated water is one of the most dangerous risks you take daily. Short-term risks include: eyes, sinus, throat, skin and lung irritation. Long-term risks include: excessive free radical formation (that ages you!), higher vulnerability to genetic mutation and cancer development; and difficulty metabolizing cholesterol that can cause hardened arteries. – Science News

ACV SHOWER MASSAGE GIVES EXTRA BODY BONUS: (in 32oz. bottle dilute 1/2 cup apple cider vinegar and water.) Pour all over body before you get out of shower. Now take thick washcloth, rub in for 3-5 minutes. When drying rub thick dry washcloth over back and then front too.

Swimming is a Great Nerve Force Builder

Swimming is one of the greatest exercises for building Nerve Force. In our lifelong study of athletic sports, we have found that swimmers have the best reserves of Nerve Force. There is something about swimming that has a relaxing effect on the whole nervous system. If either of us were President of the United States, we would have thousands of swimming pools built so that they would be available for everyone! In our opinion, swimming is definitely a great Health and Nerve Builder.

We wrote this book in beautiful Hawaii, where there is the finest ocean swimming in the world. We urge you to find a clean safe ocean, river, lake, stream or swimming pool and make swimming a part of your exercise when possible. (Wear ear plugs and eye goggles.) Don't tell us you are afraid of the water or you can't swim! It's possible to banish your fears of water and learn to swim with the help of a competent instructor.

Years ago on the beach at Waikiki we met a woman who was 78 years young. All her life, she had lived with a dread of the water and consequently could not swim. But she came to Hawaii determined to learn how to swim and banish her fears. After a few months she had accomplished both of her goals! She told us that during the greater part of her life she had been a victim of nerves and a poor sleeper. Since she learned to swim, however, her nervousness had completely disappeared and she was now sleeping like a healthy and happy newborn baby!

We urge you to make swimming a part of your life, too. You will find it a non-strenuous sport and a constant source of pleasure – as well as a great Nerve Force builder. Make use of the great health-building power of water!

Love makes the world go 'round, and it's everlasting when it's written with caring, loving advice that will improve and enrich your life! This is why my father and I love sharing with you the health wisdoms which can be with you on your long life's journey. Our books on health, fitness and longevity go 'round the world spreading health, peace of mind and love! – Patricia Bragg

Enjoy Energy from Gentle Sunbathing

All living things on earth depend on solar energy for their existence. The sun is the primary source of energy. Earth would be a barren, frigid place if it were not for the magic rays of the sun! All things that live, breathe and grow need the energy of the sun. Sun gives us light, and were it not for light, there would be no you or me. Earth would be in darkness and void of life! Mankind gains health, vitality and longevity in the gentle, healing rays of the sun.

The people who are indoors too long have sallow, ghostly-looking skin. That is why so many women hide their sun-starved skin with face makeup. People who are deprived of the vital rays of the sun have a pallid look. They are actually dying for want of solar energy! The direct rays of the gentle sun on the naked body supply vitality and dynamic energy and recharge the human storage battery with renewed strength to build powerful and vibrant Nerve Force! **Life-giving sunshine is essential to your health, happiness and longevity.**

The rays of the sun are powerful germicides. As the skin imbibes more of these rays, it stores up enormous amounts of this germ-killing energy. The gentle sun provides a remedy for the nervous person filled with anxiety, worry, stresses and strains. When these tense people get in the early morning or late afternoon gentle sunshine, its healing rays on their body give them what nerves and body are crying out for and that is relaxation!

Vitamin D3 is made when UVB light from the sun is absorbed by the skin. This is the most natural form. Learn more by reading "Vitamin D Solution" by Michael F. Holick, Ph.D., M.D., Professor Boston University and recipient of prestigious "Linus Pauling Prize" for his extensive research on Vitamin D.

Daily intake of Vitamin D of (at least 4,000 IU) are needed to reduce risk of cancers, Multiple Sclerosis and Type 1 Diabetes. Only about 10% of the U.S. population has levels in this range, mainly people who work outdoors. Sunlight is the prime source of Vitamin D. Sardines, oily fishes, mushrooms and soymilk are excellent Vitamin D sources. Check with your health care practitioner to determine your optimum Vitamin D intake.

Gentle Sunbathing Works Miracles!

When you begin sunbathing, start with short time periods until you condition your body to take more. The best time for beginners to start taking 10 and 15 minute sunbaths is in the early morning sunshine until 10 a.m. or late afternoon sunshine after 3 p.m. Between 11 and 3 we usually avoid stronger, burning rays. Please don't use sunscreens with chemicals or PABA as these chemicals are harmful. When absorbed through the skin, they disrupt our body's balanced hormone ecosystem. Use all-natural sunscreens.

The cool rays of the sun rejuvenate the skin and also help keep eyes healthy and in focus. Gentle sun is a tonic for frazzled nerves. Its cool rays calm, quiet and soothe the nerves while helping to promote a relaxed feeling. You can combine a nap with a sunbath which will help refill the body reservoirs with Nerve Force.

Enjoy Sunshine for Super Health

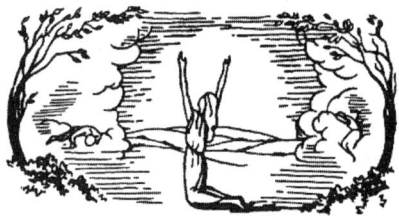

That is why my father and I have always loved the precious sunshine and why we made our main home in California, the great golden sunshine state. We have an organic farm in Santa Barbara near the ocean where we get benefits of clean air and sunshine.

Gentle sunshine is a soothing tonic, a stimulant and a Great Healer for the body, also sunshine is healthy for eyes! As you bask in the warm, gentle sunshine (not hot afternoon sun), millions of nerve endings absorb the energy from the sun and transform it so the body's nervous system can use it.

QUICK TIP: To avoid environmental toxins that overload your immune system – eat only organic foods, stop smoking and don't hang out with anyone who does and get gentle sun exposure to boost Vitamin D3 levels.

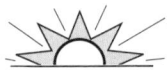

Sunshine gives energy and life to the earth, to all plants, trees and all living creatures.

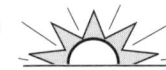

Keep Your Emotions Under Control

The Seventh Step to Building A Powerful Nerve Force

Common sense dictates that one of the first steps towards having a greater Nerve Force consists in checking the waste of the Nerve Force squandered in unnecessary emotions. When you have learned to expend less Nerve Force than your nervous system develops, this brings you more real peace and power mentally, physically, emotionally and spiritually.

Follow These Stress Reducing Guidelines:

Avoid the super-person complex! Some people want too much from themselves. They are perfectionists. They are full of tensions from pushing themselves beyond their human capacity to perform. We believe in perfection, but not at the cost of nerve exhaustion! One person cannot be skilled in everything. Do your best with those tasks which you cannot do so well and let it go at that. No one asks or expects you to accomplish the impossible, so don't demand it of yourself! You will have a much longer, healthier and happier fulfilled life.

Talk out your worries! Don't bottle everything up. If you feel you have a legitimate "beef" against someone, go to that person and quietly talk things out. Just as it takes a good storm to clear up the atmosphere when the weather is "tense," a good talk will usually clear up a disturbed emotional atmosphere. Do not harbor resentments! Get them off your chest as quickly and as calmly as possible! Nine times out of ten they arise from a misunderstanding – either on your part, the other person's or both.

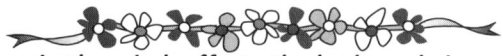

Whatever occurs in the mind, effects the body and visa versa. Mind and body cannot be considered independently. When the two are out of sync, both the emotional and physical stress can erupt.
– Hippocrates, the Father of Medicine, 400 B.C.

Communicate . . . this applies to all relationships – whether it be your mate, children, in-laws, relatives, friends or co-workers, etc. So many husbands, wives or parents and children have let resentments build up inside until they can no longer talk with one another. Sadly they built a wall out of pebbles! If you have let things get to this stage, you might be heading for a nervous breakdown! You may need to place your confidence in a good friend, therapist, relative or clergy person. Talking things over with someone who can be objective will relieve stress and enable you to view your plight clearly and help you find a logical solution to your problems.

Beware of your temper. Temper is too good a thing to lose! Under control, your temper becomes a driving force that can push you forward to the accomplishment of worthwhile goals. Out of control, your temper can destroy you, your relationships, business and others as well.

When you get irate you are wasting your Nerve Force. You are throwing away precious nerve energy. A "fit of temper" often causes nervous and physical exhaustion.

Start counting and keep on counting when you feel your temper rising. Don't say anything you will regret! Get into some vigorous physical activity at once. The best way to cool your anger is to take a brisk walk in the open air. Get away from the person or situation that is sending you into a rage. No matter how good you might feel after you "tell them off" you will lose precious Nerve Force in doing so. Swimming, gardening, housework or any other type of physical work or exercise will help work off your temper and use that Nerve Force constructively.

Don't resort to physical violence when your temper rises. The answer is not in fighting, hitting or beating! That is how crimes and murders are committed! Channel and exercise that unleashed nerve energy into constructive activities that will harm no one – yourself or anyone else. **Keep your temper under healthy control at all times!**

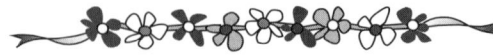

In Framingham Heart Study, women who reported suppressing their anger experienced highest rate of first heart attacks.
– FraminghamHeartStudy.org

Avoid Arguing, Teasing, Bullying & Nagging

Thousands of murders have been committed and endless hatred, bitterness and anger have resulted from heated arguments that had their beginnings in a friendly discussion of a trivial subject. An argument is a form of mental combat. We fully realize that discussions and arguments can sharpen one's wits and are often highly instructive. There are few people, however, who can indulge in friendly arguments without becoming upset! Negative excitement causes nerve strain and should be avoided by all ages, especially seniors and children. We have met hundreds of people suffering from nerve disorders which were due mainly to negative habits of nerve abuse.

The worst time in the world to get into any kind of argument is at mealtime! If there is anything that will completely upset your digestion, it's arguing when you are eating! We both believe that constant arguments at the table can bring on stomach ulcers and indigestion.

When a person with sensitive nerves – who is likely to become unduly excited – realizes that a discussion has reached a combative stage, that particular conversation should be discontinued at once.

Don't quarrel. Don't nag, bully or tease and do not permit yourself to be nagged, bullied or teased. Avoid people who do so. If you allow someone to "get your goat" they will be tempted to continue plaguing you. But if you appear impervious, ignore them or simply walk away in silence they're likely to let you alone.

There are some personalities that just don't mix well! Not everyone whom you come in contact with is going to like you or agree with your ideas! The same holds true from your point of view. Learn to live and let live! In our busy lives we've come into contact with people who irritate us. We keep out of their way and avoid them. Even with family there will be some who irritate you. Just keep your distance from them.

Before you speak ask yourself if what you are going to say is true, is kind, is necessary, is helpful. If the answer is no, maybe what you are about to say should be left unsaid. – Bernard Meltzer

Don't argue with them – it burns up precious Nerve Force! Don't try to convert them to your ideas or philosophy unless they are willing – then share a Bragg book with them or one suggested on page 66.

Don't hate these people. When you hate a person you are destroying yourself! Look upon these people as you would a bad odor – simply stay away from them! If you're forced to be in their company try to be pleasant but have as little to say to them as possible.

Shun Constant Suspicion

Many people make themselves unhappy, poison their minds and strain their nerves with extreme suspicion. They are constantly living in fear that someone is trying to cheat, rob or deceive them. They believe in the doctrine that "Everyone is a thief until proven otherwise."

This extreme suspicion may save a person a few dollars during their lifetime and may occasionally prevent them from being deceived . . . but does it pay? Is it fair toward those who are honest? We don't think so – because it wrecks one's health! Granted, you may be cheated occasionally, but we consider such money better lost than spent on nerve drugs and doctors!

Reap the Rewards of Smiling

Here's a great old wise saying, *"Laugh and the world laughs with you. Cry and you cry alone."* It has often been truly stated that the act of laughing causes certain beneficial vibrations that promote circulation in the vital abdominal region. We are also thoroughly convinced that laughing promotes health because this positive mental condition prompts laughter (see next page). Make an angry face, soon you will feel grouchy and ready to resent the slightest offense – real or fancied. This negative mental attitude depresses the nerves, and effects the heart and lungs and so on. Laughing produces the opposite – a positive effect upon your entire being! Read the classic, *Anatomy of an Illness* by Norman Cousins. This famous book reinforces these principles! Seek out happy, humorous books and videos. Also choose radio and TV programs that make you laugh and smile!

Happy Feelings Are Internal Smiles

Try this experiment. Stop reading and smile. Do you feel unaccountably happy internally, although at the moment you may not have a special reason to be happy? Now make an angry face. You will observe that you feel angry. If we placed a sphygmograph on your wrist to record your heart pulsations and blood waves, the tracings would show a decided depression in your heart action, proving that your forced grouchy attitude has caused an immediate depression of all your vital organs. So practice smiling! Smile when you read, when you are tranquil and while at rest. Smile when you are angry or worried. Eventually the smile will grow on your face and give you a happy expression! That external smile will soon give you a happy feeling inside – an internal smile!

Keep away from people who have those dark and gloomy expressions on their faces. That is one reason we like to be with young children and healthy teenagers. They laugh. There does not have to be too much to laugh at to produce their warm, natural laughter. We also like to be around people who have a good sense of humor. We love people who keep young at heart, and are kind and considerate, regardless of their calendar years! Emotions are contagious. Be around people who feel happy and you will feel happy too! Smile and almost always you will get a smile back in response.

Instant Mood Lifters

If you're feeling a little blue, have handy a list of positive actions you can take that will lift your spirits! After all, actions always speak louder – and do much more – than words.

Here are Some Tried & True Mood Builders:

Take a brisk walk. Exercise outdoors in fresh air and sunshine, it always has positive effects on your total health.

Spend time with a young child. Their simple outlook on life is a reminder that things aren't as bad as you think. Being childlike at times has merit! Enjoy your pets.

Share smiles – we shall never know all the good a simple smile can do!

Laughter does miracles! Read the cartoon (funny) pages. Childlike simplicity is refreshing. Learn to find the absurd humor in whatever is bothering you. As someone once said, "Don't take life so seriously, because you never get out of it alive anyway."

Take a moment to walk in the other persons shoes. If someone has upset you, think about the problems and sorrows in their life. This allows for some perspective on the situation and maybe some solutions.

Pretend you're happy. It sounds silly, but it works! If you smile and act happy, your body responds similarly. In many instances, being happy or content is a matter of choice. American sociologist M. Kathleen Casey says, "Pain is inevitable, suffering is optional." Much of our emotional and physical suffering can be alleviated by mind-body techniques because they are intertwined and want to heal each other. These techniques can help neutralize the stress and even the pain on our bodies.

Remove Negative Chips Off Your Shoulders

If a person says a cutting thing to you, forget it! Don't make a big issue of it and waste your vital Nerve Force arguing about it. Most mean people are usually unhealthy and mentally sick. Don't stoop down to their low level! Brush them off as you would a fly. Life is too precious to let others pull you down – and they can't unless you allow it! Many mentally sick people do try to get others down because "misery loves company." Don't join them! Avoid them! Let the other fellow hate, envy, be jealous and live a negative mental life. Not you! Be too smart to let this kind of thinking sicken you. In our long lives, we have known people who actually poisoned themselves to death with their violent hatreds! Uncontrolled emotions can make you sick, unhappy, nervous and a physical wreck.

Please stop looking for perfection in people! We all have some weaknesses and there are no 100% perfect humans. Try to see the good in people you are thrown in contact with and also in yourself!

Nothing transforms a person as much as changing from a negative attitude to a healthy positive attitude!

Paul C. Bragg Practiced Thought Substitution

My father's mother was a wise and noble woman who had a splendid philosophy to guide him. It was she who taught Dad thought substitution. He remembers it well:

"My constant companion was a little dog named Wilbur, whom I loved very dearly. One day Wilbur was killed. Heartbroken, I came to my mother with my grief. As I sobbed in her arms, she told me how to conquer the pain of my loss with thought substitution. Instead of grieving over my dog, she told me that I should change my thoughts to the happy times I had with Wilbur – such as the long hikes in the springtime when the dogwood was in bloom, or the way Wilbur used to scare a rabbit and give chase, but the rabbit would always outsmart Wilbur. Before I realized it, I was laughing through my tears as I recalled my good times with Wilbur. From then on, whenever I would think about my dog, I would automatically replace my sense of loss with a happy memory."

"Through my mother's guidance I learned to apply healthy thought substitution (visualization) when needed to heal sorrows. The substitution of happy thoughts for sad ones saved my emotional Nerve Force throughout my life! Grief over loss of a loved one is the greatest of all nerve strains. It may depress the nervous system enough to cause death. I know such grief. In spite of my positive philosophy and remarkable physical stamina, I have lost many pounds in just days through intense grief and found my vital organs, especially my heart and lungs, so depressed that I found it difficult to breathe. I know how hard it's to bring grief under control, but it can be done! ***Thought substitution is the secret."***

Having a bad day? Try walking around the block several times or run up and down a few flights of stairs. You'll return to the task at hand less troubled because the physiological changes caused by even moderate exercise calms the mind.

A good laugh is sunshine in a house. – William Makepeace Thackeray

Only one thought can occupy the mind at any one time. By an effort of will we can force out the grief-stricken, unhappy thoughts and replace them with tender, happy memories. Sorrow is a futile waste of Nerve Force. Tears cannot erase the cause of grief or emotional torment of any kind. This useless waste of nerve energy can be stopped with thought substitution (visualization). Let happy, positive thoughts occupy your mind. It all comes back to the saying ***The kingdom of heaven is within you. It's within your power to make your kingdom a wonderful, inspiring, relaxing, stress-free heaven on earth!***

Send Your Worry to the Winds

As we stated earlier in this book, worry can destroy you if you let it get the upper hand. Worry – like grief – is greatly exaggerated by many people and is employed as a means of self-torture. Many people enlarge their worries so that they may be pitied and petted – a selfish practice.

It's true worry is often unavoidable, like war. We can't always turn our backs upon it, especially if it means business ruin, loss of love and poverty. But we can always use clear thinking, common sense and good judgment to our advantage! We should bar worry from our minds since we know little can be gained by it. On the contrary, the more we worry, the greater the strain on our Nerve Force and the less able we are to overcome our troubles. We should remain optimistic in the face of all obstacles! Remember it is always the positive optimist who succeeds, never the negative pessimist!

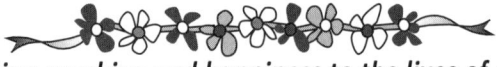

Those who bring sunshine and happiness to the lives of others cannot keep it from themselves. – James Matthew Barrie, Peter Pan Creator

---

Be mindful of what quarreling feels like in your body, emotions and thoughts. A regular diet of quarreling is not good for your long-term physical and mental health. It takes two to quarrel and only one to stop it.

A Harvard Study shows that men with the highest anger on personality tests are three times more likely to develop heart disease. High blood pressure affects 1 in 3 of all adults in the U.S.; it is often called "the silent killer".

Cheerfulness is the atmosphere under which all things thrive. – Richter

Make Your Own Sunshine & Happiness

Some people's cheerfulness and joy is governed by the weather. When the sun shines brightly, they are bright. When the weather is gloomy, they're gloomy. There are more suicides in gloomy weather than when it's sunny!

Try the smiling cure. Learn to love the rain when it rains, love darkness when it is dark and love the blazing heat when it is blazing hot. **James Whitcomb Riley wrote**:

It is not any use to grumble and complain;
It's just as cheap and easy to rejoice;
When God sorts out the weather
and sends the rain,
Then, rain is my choice.

Singing in the Rain is one of our favorite songs. When you are healthy and happy the weather doesn't bother you. Your disposition is not governed by the barometer. You can make your own sunshine within yourself!!!

Have an Attitude of Gratitude!

Gratitude creates happiness because it makes us feel full and complete. Gratitude is the realization that we have everything we need! One of the truths about gratitude is that it's impossible to feel both the positive emotion of thankfulness and a negative emotion such as anger or fear at the same time. Gratitude gives only positive feelings – love, compassion, joy, and hope. As we focus on what we are thankful for, fear, anger, and bitterness and unhappy thoughts simply melt away. – Excerpt from *Attitudes of Gratitude* by M.J. Ryan

Little acts of kindness throughout the day will make your life so much better and bring a little sunshine to others along the way.

Wherever you go, no matter what the weather, always bring your own sunshine. – Anthony J. D'Angelo

Living in harmony with the universe is living totally alive, full of vitality, health, joy, inner peace, power, love, and abundance on every level. – Shakti Gawain

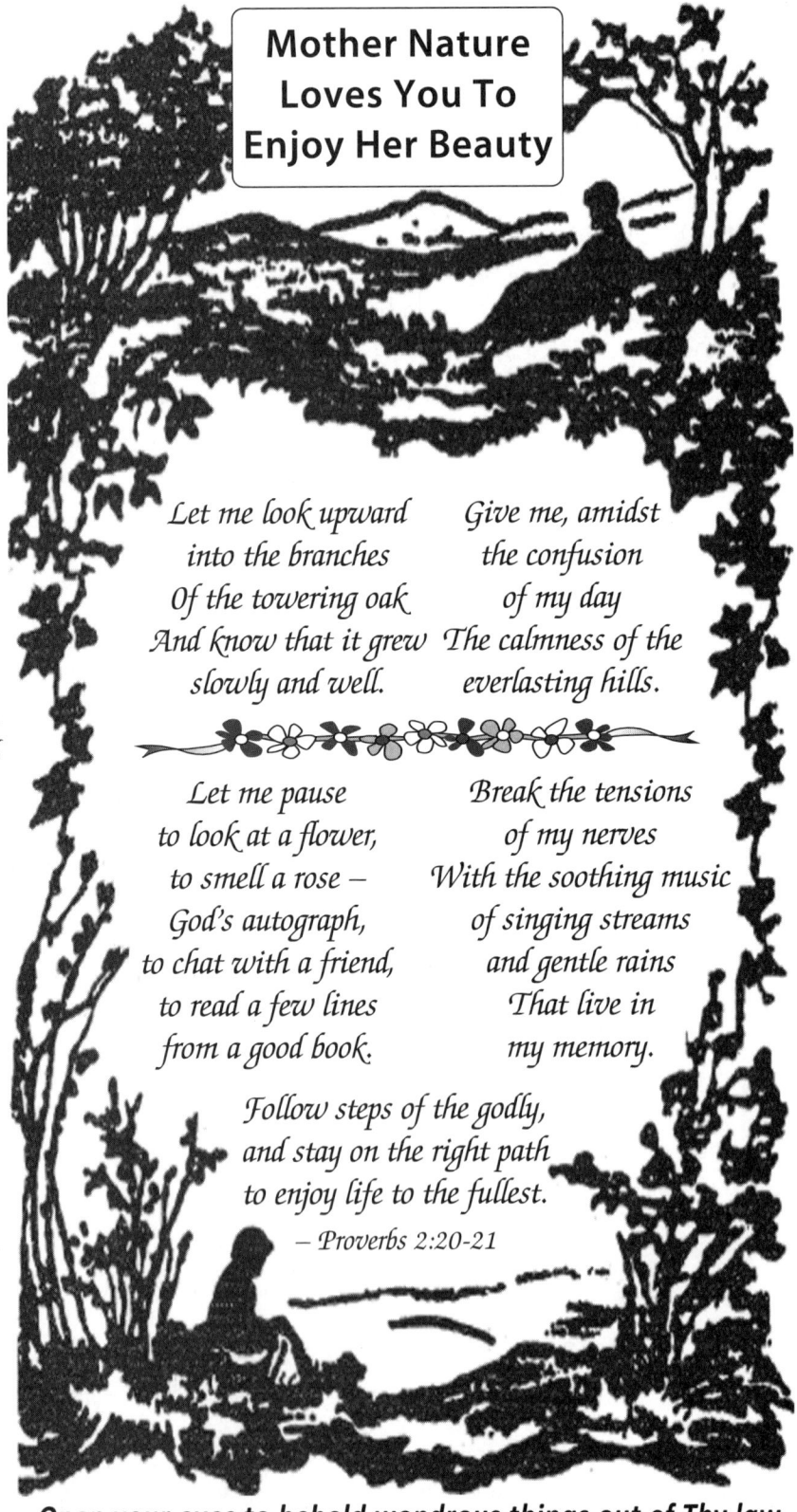

Mother Nature Loves You To Enjoy Her Beauty

Let me look upward
into the branches
Of the towering oak
And know that it grew
slowly and well.

Give me, amidst
the confusion
of my day
The calmness of the
everlasting hills.

Let me pause
to look at a flower,
to smell a rose –
God's autograph,
to chat with a friend,
to read a few lines
from a good book.

Break the tensions
of my nerves
With the soothing music
of singing streams
and gentle rains
That live in
my memory.

Follow steps of the godly,
and stay on the right path
to enjoy life to the fullest.
– Proverbs 2:20-21

Open your eyes to behold wondrous things out of Thy law.
– Psalm 119:18

Healthy Relaxation: How to Relax the Nerves

The Eighth Step to Building A Powerful Nerve Force

The word "relax" is very much like the word "love." When you ask the average person what it means to relax, you get all kinds of different answers – just as you do when you ask for a definition of love.

We would often hear people say at our athletic club, "I want to smoke a cigarette and relax." For others it's whiskey and soda, a cup of coffee, tea or an ice cold cola. None of these people have the slightest idea what the word relax means! They are all talking about stimulants! It is impossible to relax when you are pouring alcohol, tobacco, coffee, tea and cola drinks into your system. This is the opposite of relaxing. This is whipping your nerves with powerful unhealthy drug stimulants.

Let's get the correct definition of the word relax and then we will carry on from there. Webster's dictionary says, ***Relax: to make less tense or rigid; to become less intense or severe; to cast off social restraint, nervous tension or anxiety; to seek rest or recreation.*** We think these definitions are the correct meaning of the word relax. You cannot relax in the true sense of the word when you use stimulants and powerful drugs. We'll admit that stimulants and drugs will deaden the nerves for a time. You can give a person a powerful sedative and it will temporarily calm them, or – in many cases – knock a person out cold. Some sedatives will put a person into a deep stupor, but it is impossible to say that these people are relaxed – their body and mind are drugged!

Caffeine: Increases blood pressure, depletes calcium and magnesium from body, elevates cholesterol levels and increases level of dangerous homocysteine in blood. When your coffee high wears off, you feel the drop in terms of fatigue, irritability, headache and confusion.
– "Caffeine Blues" by Stephen Cherniske, M.S.

People use the word relax very carelessly. Some will tell you they are going on a trip to relax and get away from all the tensions of their lives. While this may help relieve daily stress, bad habits of living are carried along. We will admit that a trip can refresh you – but true relaxation comes from removing bad lifestyle habits!!!

Relaxation is a Healthy, Soothing Feeling

Relaxation is a special feeling. There is no other way to express it. This feeling is not something you can turn off and on at will. Relaxation is something that must be built up in the conscious and subconscious mind, something you build up in every one of the billions of cells in your body, in your entire nervous system, in your vital organs and in your muscles.

There have been times – yes, many times – when you have correctly let your feelings direct your life. Haven't you said to yourself more than once, "I have a feeling I should not go on that trip as I planned to do?" Let's say it was to be a plane trip. So you listened to the inner voice of your feelings and did not go. Then something came up in your life that made you glad you didn't go. You relied upon your wise guidance and your feelings.

We have often said, "I have a feeling that person doesn't like me." Sure enough, we find that person is trying to undermine our character to others. Or, someone hurts you dreadfully and you say to them, "You have hurt my feelings." You feel the hurt deep inside.

Yes, we do have feelings and we do feel things. Relaxation is a feeling. Your feelings allow your nerves to relax. Your feelings can banish stress, strain and tensions to bring calm, inner peace and serenity. Feeling is the life force within you that is always working for you. All it needs is a chance. It is astonishing how few people get their physical, mental and emotional debris out of the way and let their wise feelings work for them.

The greatest discovery of my generation is that human beings can alter their lives by altering their attitudes of mind. – William James (1842-1920)

Where your focus goes – your energy flows!

In times of stress be bold, strong and valiant. – Horace, 65 B.C.

Everyone knows what it is to feel *miserable* . . . just as everyone knows how it feels to be tired, exhausted, weak, sad or depressed. All people know what pain feels like. Our feelings don't deceive us. We all know how we feel when we get up in the morning. We know how we feel during the day. **Feelings are a vital part of our lives!**

If we feel nervous, weak, tired and miserable we produced those feelings with our incorrect daily living habits. Feeling follows the law of cause and effect. Every effect in life is produced by a cause. You get out of life just what you put into it. It is one of the great and inflexible laws of life. Most people are plagued with stress, strains and tensions. These conditions do not just appear out of a blue sky! They are motivated by a cause.

Relaxation is a feeling produced by one's actions, attitude and environment. If you follow a defined program of building Nerve Force, you can produce the feeling of complete relaxation! However, you must earn this feeling. There is no use trying to get it with a cigarette, cup of coffee, tea, cola or an alcoholic drink.

Feelings, Tension and Relaxation Create the Heartbeat of Life

As you obey and live by the Laws of Mother Nature you'll automatically earn the right to relax when your body needs relaxation! There is nothing wrong with tension. Tension is part of life. For example – when we have walked out onto the platform to lecture before 5,000 people for two hours we were bound to feel some tension! Life is movement and movement requires tension as well as release. How is that fact expressed in your body?

You have a miraculous organ in your chest cavity that is active from the moment it begins to function before birth to the instant of your death. That miracle muscular organ is your heart. How does it keep going for so many years? Study it closely. Observe exactly how it works. It tenses and then relaxes, tenses and relaxes. Thus it can go on and on and on. There is a great lesson for us here.

Open your mind for the doors of wisdom are never shut! – Ben Franklin

---

Be kind to your heart – it takes care of you and keeps you alive!!!

The heart is like life itself. It should be made up of tension and relaxation. To get a task done – whether it is large or small – we must draw upon our Nerve Force reserves. We put an extra push into our efforts and this extra push is tension. If our nerves are healthy and we are working correctly, when the effort of the task is over we should automatically have the feeling of relaxation.

You can't force relaxation any more than you can change the beating of your heart. Relaxation is a feeling, always remember that. It is something that works naturally within your nervous system. Live by Mother Nature's Laws and you will never have to worry about relaxation. This feeling will come to you naturally.

Pay no attention to people who tell you to relax, unless they also tell you how to tense for action and how to coordinate the two states. Life is ebb and flow. It's part of life to tense when necessary – and then to relax! We have heard lecturers tell students to "let go"– to lie in bed and raise a leg, then drop it and tell the leg it is completely relaxed. Do the same with an arm. These are good exercises, but true relaxation takes more than exercise. **Relaxation is a beautiful soothing feeling within your body and mind.**

Strive to make your nervous system so powerful that your body will automatically shift from tension to relaxation. This will be your natural rhythm of living if you earn it by healthful living. It is the great law of compensation at work. Under the wise Laws of Mother Nature you only get what you earn. There is a price tag for everything in your life. You get absolutely nothing for nothing. You must earn the feeling of true relaxation. You cannot get it with artificial chemicals.

Be good to your body and it will be good to you! Abuse the body and it will punish you with tension, stress, strain, even constipation! The Laws of Mother Nature don't punish you – you punish yourself! Live so that the feeling of relaxation will come to you when it's needed. Be a friend to yourself! Treat yourself right so you can enjoy a long, healthy and relaxed life! *The kingdom of heaven is within.* When your body is completely relaxed then you will experience an inner serenity and the true joy of peaceful living.

There Are No Magic Cures

No drug exists that will build Nerve Force. All the artificial stimulants such as coffee, tea, tobacco, colas, alcohol and drugs are in a low rate of vibration. These will dissipate, drain and damage your Nerve Force, not build it. Yes, there are drugs that will push or quiet your nerves such as pep pills, which so many nervous people use daily to keep them going. There are drugs that will stun and quiet the nerves when they are unmanageable. But no conscientious health practitioner will prescribe these drugs except when absolutely necessary to tide a patient over during a crisis.

There are no magic, quick cures for people who have exhausted their Nerve Force that will build Nerve Force or "tone up" the body and its many functions. Nutritional supplements and herbs and Chiropractic, massages, exercise and special baths are all valuable therapies, but only as local treatments. **Only you can strike at the root of nerve or functional weaknesses by your lifestyle – how you live and the way you think!**

There is only one sure way to have powerful Nerve Force . . . you must build it by adopting a constructive program of living. We wish there were shortcuts we could recommend to you. We are all controlled by the law of compensation. You get nothing for nothing. To build powerful Nerve Force, you must work at it each day of your life. It is through knowledge and wisdom that we achieve the good things in life. **It is through positive thinking and positive action that we build supreme, awesome vitality and super Nerve Force. Start now!**

Ten Little, Two-Letter Words of Action To Say Daily:

If it is to be, it is up to me!

Free yourself from bondage of these killing habits:

- "I will not use tobacco."
- "I will not over-eat."
- "I will not drink black tea."
- "I will not use salt."
- "I will not drink coffee, sodas and alcoholic drinks."
- "I will not clog my arteries with saturated fats."

Be your own Health Captain and do what needs to be done for your health!

Ten Great No-Calorie Stress Busters:

1. Turn on your favorite music and dance.
2. Enroll in a yoga class, or take Tai chi, Qi gong, Pilates or stretching class.
3. Call a good friend and have some laughs.
4. Read inspiring Bragg books and health magazines.
5. Take a hot herbal bubble bath or vinegar bath.
6. Go to the gym or take a brisk fresh air walk.
7 Get a massage – best at your home when possible.
8. Write and release your feelings in your daily journal.
9. Watch an inspiring movie, comedy or travelogue.
10. Close your eyes, relax, do 'yoga breathing' – breathe in slowly through nose, letting air fill lungs completely down to the diaphragm. Hold in briefly, then exhale through the mouth slowly. See: *HealthAndYoga.com.*

The Benefits of Full Yoga Breathing

- Helps release acute and chronic muscular tensions in the body, especially around the heart and digestive organs.
- Increases lung capacity – this helps asthma and emphysema sufferers overcome fear of having shortness of breath attacks.
- Encourages proper nervous stimulus to cardiovascular system.
- Dramatically reduces emotional and nervous anxiety.
- Helps detox by increasing carbon dioxide & oxygen exchange.
- Helps auto-immune system by increased energy to endocrine system that regulates metabolism, tissue function, internal temperature, water balance, ions and your personality moods.
- Calms the mind and integrates mental and physical balance.
- Contributes to vitality, energy and relaxation.

As often as possible make yourself smile and laugh; it opens the blood vessels in the back of your head to physically lift your mood. Choose to be happy in spite of circumstances. You can make yourself happy, it's your inner Nerve Force and attitude that sparkles from within.

DANCING HELPS YOUR HEART: A study has found that dancing has the same benefit for heart patients as working out at the gym. Hit the dance floor and help your heart said readersdigest.com. "I love dancing! I've danced the Polka on the TV show with Lawrence Welk. I danced with Fred Astaire, Gene Kelly, Bob Hope and Arthur Murray."

Enjoy Life!

The Ninth Step to Building A Powerful Nerve Force

Learn to Live Joyously with Yourself

Remember you came into this world alone and leave it alone. It's nice to have a good family, friends and a mate, but – above all – you must learn to love living with yourself! Don't become too intimate with too many people because "familiarity often breeds contempt". Maintain a high personal dignity level, even with yourself. You must be good company for yourself! We have never been bored in our lives. We go on nature hikes and get to understand ourselves better. As we grow to understand ourselves better, we get to understand other humans more.

Lead a busy, happy, creative life. If you follow our Nerve Force Building Program, you are going to be busy! You will have a happy, well-rounded, balanced day with your meditation and prayer, your exercises and deep breathing, healthy eating program and reading new, instructive books, plus continuing with your daily work. A busy person is a happy person with little time to worry. Life becomes a great adventure. Enjoy every minute of it! We only get 24 precious hours a day. No one gets more – be they king, queen or billionaire. So live each day as though it were your last! Make every minute count! Time is too precious to waste! When someone says, "I have to kill time, I'm bored," we think, "How sad!" **Now, accept new challenges. Don't be afraid to tackle any job or chore, no matter how big! Get going and start living healthy and successfully now!**

Slow Down and Enjoy Each Day!

Life has lots of simple things to enjoy. But if you move too fast, you might overlook them! Don't be in such a hurry. Look at the world around you. Notice the grass, the flowers, the sunrise and sunset – Mother Nature is all around you. Take time to pause, to see and enjoy!

Healthy Body = More Peaceful Mind

Everyone feels happier when they are looking good and taking a multi vitamin and mineral supplement. They contribute specifically to your health and looks!

- **Vitamin D** contributes to the strength and density of bones. A lack of vitamin D can lead to osteoporosis, which often affects the posture, a reason seniors do better with some "vitamin D3's sunshine" and a good multi-mineral with calcium, boron and magnesium. Also get 15 minutes of gentle sun exposure a few times a week, preferably early or late sun (see pages 141-142).

- **Vitamin A** contributes to healthy skin, hair, eyes and strong, durable bones and strong tooth enamel.

- **The B vitamins** – niacin, riboflavin, B6, B12 and also magnesium help to prevent growth retardation in young people. Niacin and riboflavin help prevent skin rashes, lip sores and lip cracks and protects your nerves.

- **Vitamin B complex** promotes normal functioning of your brain, nerves and helps in resistance to stress.

- **Folic acid** plays a vital role in the smooth functioning of a healthy body, it improves brain function, helps lessen depression, anxiety and lowers homocysteine levels. In addition to supplements, folic acid is found in dates and broccoli (page 84-85).

- **Vitamin C** (and Ester C) is a powerful antioxidant which fights diseases, colds, flu, etc. (including cancer) and helps prevent high blood pressure and blood clotting. It's vital for tissue growth and repair (especially bruising). It also helps reduce cholesterol levels and increases the absorption of the mineral iron.

All vitamins and minerals listed above and many more which are found naturally in The Bragg Healthy Lifestyle Diet will help you maintain a healthier, happier body and a more peaceful mind, so you can enjoy life more!

Don't forget to MOVE! The body is a magnificent machine and exercise is vital to lasting health! There are many options you can enjoy by yourself or with family or friends: walking, biking, dancing, hiking, tennis, swimming, etc. Just remember to Enjoy Life!

The Biochemistry of Mental Health

Having spent much of our lifetimes in the research and practical application of the biochemical relationship between nutrition and human health – and for much of that time having felt like "a voice in the wilderness" – we are happy to have lived long enough to see our Bragg teachings being verified by medical research. For years we have warned people around the world that the increased devitalization and "embalming" of foodstuffs consumed by the general public would result in an alarming increase in cancers, premature death and in mental and physical deficiencies among adults and children! Three generations now show the effects of being reared on this "junk food" diet and its dramatic increase in hyperactive and violent youngsters.

Nervous Problems Are Epidemic!

In our hectic world there is often so much pressure to stay on the go that we forget how to relax. We've met many people over the years who never took time to slow down and smell the roses! These people never take breaks from their stressful lives until it's too late – working, rushing and worrying until their health deteriorates.

It's no wonder that modern medicine is reporting epidemics in nervous disorders. Medical conditions like Attention Deficit Hyperactivity Disorders (ADHD) and Chronic Fatigue Syndrome (CFS), which were almost unheard of in the past, are now common diagnoses. In fact, according to The National Institute of Mental Health, there are over 17 million Americans suffering from ADHD alone and 4 million ADHD victims are children! Sad Facts!!!

Happiness is not being pained in body or troubled in mind.
– Thomas Jefferson, 3rd U.S. President, 1797-1801

It's magnificent to live long if one keeps healthy, youthful and active.
– Harry Emerson Fosdick, American Clergyman (1878-1969)

Nutritional Therapy Brings Miracles For Hyperactive and Challenged Children

Even more than the non-responsive "challenged" child, the hyperkinetic slow learner or "hyperactive under-achiever" is becoming a more common serious problem today. These children are characterized by almost continuous irrational behavior, very short attention spans and difficulty in comprehension. A number of research studies report that children in both categories are now responding with great improvement with nutritional supplement therapy. Most notable are efforts of the New York Institute for Child Development (with a record of more than 1,500 cases) and – in San Francisco – at the Kaiser-Permanente Hospital's Allergy Clinic, the famous study directed by Dr. Benjamin Feingold (see web: *www.Feingold.org).* An individualized health program of diet and exercise is prescribed after a series of biochemical and neurological tests.

Here is Dr. Feingold's Basic Health Program:

1. Elimination of all refined sugar, refined flour products and all foods containing toxic additives, caffeine, preservatives and artificial sweeteners and coloring.
2. High protein (preferably vegetarian), low carbohydrate meals with an emphasis on fresh, raw organic fruits, vegetables and their fresh juices.
3. Natural vitamin and mineral food supplements – especially B6 and the other B vitamins, vitamin C, E, niacin, pantothenic acid, magnesium and calcium – plus others determined for the patient's needs.

In other words, this is basically the same nutritional program we have been advocating for four generations! The same diet – combined with generous doses of vitamins and minerals – is being used successfully in the treatment of children with serious brain damage at the Institute for the Achievement of Human Potential in Philadelphia, PA.

The doctor of the future will no longer treat the human frame with drugs, but rather will cure and prevent disease with nutrition.
– Thomas Edison, 1847-1931

In Dr. Feingold's research and writings he showed two companion graphs covering the ten year study that demonstrated the parallel between the yearly sales of artificial sweeteners (such as aspartame, NutraSweet, etc., see page 174), and soft drinks and the increase of hyperkinesia (hyperactivity), anger and learning difficulties among children in the United States.

About Chronic Fatigue Syndrome – CFS

CFS, is a condition in which fatigue and tiredness rule the heart and minds of its victims. These people live at a low rate of vibration which makes their normal life seem a burden. When life's small tasks become great exertions, what then are life's challenges? Clearly, chronic fatigue is a quality of life destroyer that must be understood and overcome.

Back in the 1980's, CFS was called the "Yuppie Flu," a relatively rare condition that affected mostly the upper middle class. Researchers (*SolveCFS.org*), have shattered that image. They found as many as 1 million people nationwide may suffer from CFS, and it's about 2-4 times as common in women as men, and strikes people from every age, racial, ethnic and socioeconomic group.

What Causes CFS? Scientists don't know exactly what causes Chronic Fatigue Syndrome. It may be a combination of factors. Some factors that have been studied are: *Immune System problems, Hormonal imbalances* and *Viral Infections* (suspicious viruses include Epstein-Barr virus, human herpes virus 6 and mouse leukemia viruses, without conclusive links being found).

What are the symptoms of CFS? The most common symptoms are: debilitating fatigue, impairment of short-term memory or concentration, sore throat, tender lymph nodes, muscle and joint pain, headaches, unrefreshing sleep and fatigue lasting more than 24 hours following exertion. To be diagnosed with CFS, a person must have had these symptoms for more than six months and not be diagnosed with any other medical illness or ailments. Many CFS patients are unable to hold jobs, attend school or care for their family.

There is truth in the saying that man becomes what he eats. – Gandhi

CFS Healing Testimony for The Bragg Healthy Lifestyle

Diagnosed with Chronic Fatigue Syndrome, fibromyalgia, clinical and manic depression, I have been on every drug imaginable and tried every doctor-type treatment recommended – but only got worse! In the last 6-8 months I changed my diet, began exercising and discontinued ALL medications. I have been living The Bragg Healthy Lifestyle including a weekly 24-hour fast. I feel incredible – sinus headaches and bloating gone. I am more focused and directed. Depression, fatigue, body tension – all gone! I have my life back – I am in control of my health and life! I got back to basics with the Bragg health books and healthy lifestyle. Patricia, you truly are a crusading angel and make such a difference in so many people's lives. God bless you – thank you! – Marilyn, CA

Dr. James Balch's Health Suggestions to Combat Chronic Fatigue Syndrome*:

- **Eat a well-balanced, natural, healthy diet** of 50% raw, organically grown foods and fresh "live" juices. The diet should consist mostly of fruits, vegetables, whole grains, plus raw nuts, seeds, skinless turkey and some deep-water fish. These quality foods supply nutrients that renew energy and help build your immunity.
- **Add some form of acidophilus to your diet**, and regularly consume soured products like soy yogurt, sauerkraut, yogurt, kefir, etc. Many people with chronic fatigue syndrome also are infected with candida. Acidophilus helps to keep candida under control.
- **Drink distilled water** – at least 8 glasses per day, plus freshly made fruit and vegetable juices. Water flushes out toxins and helps reduce muscle and joint pain.
- **Do not eat shellfish, fried foods, junk foods,** processed refined foods, sugar and white flour products – desserts, bread and pasta, and stay away from stimulants – coffee, black tea and cola drinks – see *Foods to Avoid List* on page 94.

Dr. James Balch, in "Prescription for Nutritional Healing" states: CFS can cause serious damage to your immune system. You must combat it.

- **Add ample fiber to your diet** and make sure that your bowels move daily (see page 41).
- **Take chlorophyll** in liquid or tablet form and take protein supplements or powders from a vegetable source such as Spirulina or Barley Green.
- **Certain amino acids may be beneficial** for those with CFS, they include: tyrosine, leucine, isoleucine, valine, lysine and taurine.
- **Get plenty of rest.** Make sure you don't over-exert yourself. Melatonin is helpful for promoting restful sleep. Skullcap and valerian root also improve sleep.
- **Try a variety of teas** from burdock root, dandelion, red clover and Pau d'Arco which help promote healing.
- **Ginkgo biloba, St. John's Wort and SAMe** are also beneficial for those with Chronic Fatigue Syndrome.
- **Taking echinacea and goldenseal enhances immune** function and helps with cold and flu symptoms.
- **Other important vitamins & nutrients are:** CoQ10, calcium, lecithin, potassium, malic acid, magnesium, manganese, vitamins A, B, C, E, zinc, garlic, black currant, primrose oil capsules, and maitake or shiitake reishi mushrooms available fresh or dried (soak 1/2 hour before eating) or in caps and powders.

For more on Chronic Fatigue Syndrome see web: *SolveCFS.org*

Avoiding Metabolic Syndrome

Metabolic Syndrome is regarded as a collection of disease risk factors caused by insulin resistance, which pre-disposes you to diabetes, heart disease and stroke. A recent study (*mercola.com*) has found a correlation between the lack of micronutrients such as folate, zinc and vitamins B12, C, E and D. To boost your metabolism, it is important to eliminate sugar and excess salt in your meals; exercise regularly and get adequate amounts of sleep.

Some therapies tried by people with CFS include: massage therapy, acupuncture, chiropractic therapy, self-hypnosis, and therapeutic touch. People with CFS may feel better with such techniques, but these therapies should be combined with an individualized exercise program that includes stretching and yoga. – see web: eMedicineHealth.com

Your biological rhythm of sleeping and awaking is known as circadian rhythm – this is intricately tied to your metabolism. If you deprive yourself of adequate sleep, you disrupt your metabolism. Lack of sleep also affects your levels of leptin and ghrelin – two hormones linked with appetite and eating. When you are sleep deprived, your body decreases production of leptin, the hormone that tells your brain that you are not hungry. At the same time, it increases your levels of ghrelin – a hormone that triggers hunger! This results in a weak and sluggish metabolism. The right amount of sleep is based on your own individual needs. See pages 63-76.

Diet is Vital to Developing Intelligence and Brain Cells

To prove that proper nutrition is effective not only for restoring normality to children with brain dysfunctions, but also for increasing learning abilities of children considered normal, New York Institute for Child Development tested the effect of controlled foods and vitamins on children in Harlem nurseries. There was a 20% increase in their I.Q.'s over 1 year! Similar studies in other parts of the country have also confirmed these findings. For example, a psychological study by Dr. M. B. Stoch and Prof. P. M. Smythe, compared undernourished children with properly nourished children from similar backgrounds and parentage, discovered a 22 I.Q. points difference in favor of the well nourished children over a period of years!

"All the learning opportunities in the world will be of no avail, unless infants are at the same time furnished with everything they need to build up their brain cell structures," states Roger J. Williams in *Nutrition Against Disease*. He also stresses that the brain is strongly vulnerable to malnutrition and its effects. **In 1998 the Salk Institute in La Jolla, CA, found in their landmark study that humans can generate new brain cells (see: *www.salk.edu*).**

Exercising, along with some weight training, eating a healthy diet, getting some healthy, gentle sunshine, and solid sleeping habits can go a long way toward optimizing your metabolism.

These studies all focus on the harmful food additives, white flour and excessive sugar, as the primary culprits that upset the normal functioning of the brain. These, of course, are the basic ingredients of "junk food" diets that most young Americans are raised on; empty calorie foodless foods. All the essential nourishment, including vitamins, minerals and other nutrients, have been "refined" out. No so-called "enrichment" with synthetic vitamins can replace natural, healthy nutrition. Dr. Feingold pointed out, some of the most harmful toxic additives are now being used in synthetic vitamins, especially in those brands widely advertised for children!

Biochemical tests on hyperactive children show they suffer from vitamin, mineral, and enzyme deficiencies and imbalances and from hypoglycemia. It's ironic that hypoglycemia (low blood sugar), is most often caused by over-eating refined white sugar and white flour products which are converted into empty calories in the body.

This excessive amount of sugar over-stimulates the production of insulin as a result of the natural biochemical reaction to rid the body of excess sugar, but the empty sugar calories are so quickly consumed that the extra insulin then depletes the body's natural sugar as well. This causes blood sugar to drop below normal, which creates an appetite for even more sugar! Unless the hypoglycemic's diet is controlled, this vicious circle keeps on repeating itself.

The brain suffers from low blood sugar more than any other part of the body. Although other organs can derive energy from various sources, the brain depends almost exclusively on the oxidation of glucose (the energy substance of sugar). Hypoglycemia starves the brain, and when you starve the brain, you starve the control "computer" center of the individual human being!

DIABETES AND BRAIN DAMAGE: New research has found people who develop diabetes and high blood pressure in middle age are more likely to have brain cell loss and other damage to the brain, as well as problems with memory and thinking skills. "In particular, diabetes has adverse effects regardless of age at which diabetes develops," says Dr. Rosebud Roberts, member of American Academy of Neurology. – webMD.com

Vitamins & Minerals to Treat Mental Issues

The biochemical-nutritional approach is making headway in that last frontier of medicine: mental illness. Many leading psychiatrists today are convinced that a physical cause can be found for various mental disorders and diseases. **Since 1959, the Brain Research Institute at UCLA has worked intensively to analyze the biochemistry of depression and other mental illnesses to discover the effect of dietary deficiencies on mental health and how these can be corrected. Amazing results are happening *(bri.ucla.edu)*.**

Dr. Carl C. Pfeiffer at the N.J. Psychiatric Institute, had found that one form of schizophrenia (known as "mauve-positive") responds to treatment with specific vitamin and mineral food supplements. He reported on the case of a 15-year-old schizophrenic patient who has been returned to, and maintained normalcy for 2 years, on daily supplements of 1,000 mgs of vitamin B6, and some zinc and manganese. When these supplements were discontinued in a test, the patient relapsed into her schizophrenic state (convulsions, insomnia, etc.). Moving forward in situations which caused stress, she simply increased her daily quota of B6 (500 to 800 mgs)! There are other reports of similar cases that responded to massive supplements of B6, and niacin (B3).

"Medicine treats symptoms, while nutrition treats causes!"

– declared by Dr. Grace Song Line, a nutritional therapy pioneer who dramatically demonstrated this principal early in her career. A native of Korea, she came to the United States after obtaining her medical degree in Japan. In 1929 she became the first woman in the U.S. to receive a degree as Doctor of Public Health. At the Michigan State Mental Hospital, Dr. Line took over the treatment of a "hopeless" case – a 20 year old girl who was unable to eat or take care of herself in any way and was being milk-fed by tube. Dr. Line stopped the milk-feeding and the electric shock treatments to which the girl had been subjected. She then put the patient on condensed liver broth supplemented by massive doses of niacinamide, plus other natural multi-vitamins and minerals fed to her through the tube, as well as a daily intravenous injection of vital B-Complex, niacinamide B3 and B12. Amazingly, within a week the girl was taking care of herself (dressing, combing her hair, etc.), had developed a normal appetite and could feed herself. The doctors at the hospital pronounced it "miraculous."

Dr. Line continued such "miracles" using nutritional therapy throughout a lifetime of treating degenerative diseases in patients of all ages. Along with therapeutic doses of supplemental vitamins and minerals, she insisted on a diet of strictly organic, chemical-free foods and pure water!

Magnesium – Essential for Healthy Nerves

The vital role of magnesium in the treatment of certain emotional and mental disorders – ranging from mental fatigue to frightening hallucinations – was not detected until very recently because magnesium levels are usually measured by sampling the blood serum. Two physicians – Dr. Richard C. W. Hall of the U.S. Naval Hospital in Orlando, Florida and Dr. Joy R. Joffe of Johns Hopkins University College of Medicine – have discovered that blood serum levels can remain normal while magnesium levels in the brain and cerebrospinal fluid may be dangerously low. This discovery has clarified previous confusion in attempts to correlate magnesium deficiency with a variety of symptoms that indicate degeneration of nerve, brain and heart tissue. Today these complications – which often appear in connection with certain conditions such as alcoholism, severe burns, chronic diarrhea, malnutrition in infants and adults, arrhythmia – are being treated successfully with magnesium orotate or sulfate, given orally or by injection.

For fast-acting relief, try slowing down. – Lily Tomlin, comedian

Natural vitamins, minerals and food supplements are good insurance factors in helping to keep the body well nourished, peaceful and healthy.

Magnesium is a superstar nutrient that plays an important role in over 300 vital functions in the body. – Life Extension Magazine (lef.org)

To assure the healthy functioning of your nerves and brain, be sure to include good sources of organic magnesium, such as nuts of all kinds (raw is best), non-hydrogenated peanut and nut butters, organic steel-cut oatmeal, raw sesame seeds, soybeans, stone-ground cornmeal, whole wheat flour, organic spinach, avocados, beans and especially raw wheat germ in your diet.

75% of Adults Deficient in Magnesium

A report by the World Health Organization found that 75% of adult Americans were eating less than the RDA (Recommended Dietary Allowance) of magnesium. **They also found that magnesium consumption tends to decrease with age.** ***"Magnesium deficiency is a concern for all ages, but for the elderly, it could be particularly serious,"*** says Richard Rivlin, M.D., Chief Nutrition Division of New York Hospital – Cornell Medical Center (*MedicalNewsToday.com*)

Magnesium is one of the body's major electrolytes, along with potassium, calcium and sodium. It is involved in over 300 enzymatic reactions in the body, and is vital for the proper functioning of the heart and nervous system. Causes for magnesium depletion include: use of birth control pills, excessive use of alcohol, a diet of refined foods and stress! Researchers believe that stress causes magnesium to be released from the cells and then excreted in the urine. Many health practitioners have found that supplementing with magnesium, rather than prescribing tranquilizers, is what is needed for those who suffer from this nervousness, restless leg syndrome, ADHD, irritability, anxiety, or depression. Studies also showed that, along with magnesium (orotate or sulfate is best), that also vitamin B6 helps ease symptoms of premenstrual syndrome.

Take 1,000 mgs of calcium daily in conjunction with 500 mgs of magnesium daily. Postmenopausal women are advised to take 1,500 mgs calcium. Choose a calcium formula that contains mixed compounds such as citrate, carbonate, aspartate and gluconate in combination with similar magnesium complex. – see: healthydirections.com

---

May food be your medicine. The natural healing force within us is the greatest force in getting well. – Hippocrates, Father of Medicine, 400 B.C.

How Much Magnesium Do You Need?

RDA for magnesium is 350 mgs for men and 300 mgs for women. Pregnant or nursing women require an extra 150 mgs. Though magnesium naturally occurs in most raw foods, a healthy daily 350 mgs is hard to attain eating processed and junk S.A.D. foods. Eat organic apples, apricots, avocados, bananas, green leafy vegetables, garlic, beans, soybeans, soy products, raw nuts and seeds, brown rice, tofu, whole wheat and other whole grains, which are rich in magnesium. Herbs such as cayenne, alfalfa, fennel, hops and paprika also add magnesium.

Only 25% of Americans consume the Recommended Daily Allowance (RDA) amount. Mildred Seelig, M.D., has spent years researching magnesium and is a renowned world authority on the subject. Dr. Seelig recommends an intake of at least 6 mg per kilogram of body weight. This would mean 300 mg for a 100-pound person, 420 mg for a 154-pound person, and 540 mg for a 200-pound person. Dr. Shari Lieberman, suggested that the optimal daily allowance for both men and women should be 500 – 750 mg daily. People with osteoporosis, high blood pressure, arrhythmia or angina, or women taking oral contraceptives, should take even higher levels, said Dr. Lieberman. Magnesium supplementing should be properly balanced to include correct levels of calcium, zinc and potassium. Robert K. Rude, M.D., Director of Bone and Mineral Clinic of Orthopedic Hospital in Los Angeles, found that magnesium deficiency is associated with low blood levels of calcium and potassium. Dr. Rude says that magnesium should be used in lower amounts cautiously by those that have impaired kidney function.

Calcium: The Other Half of the Dynamic Duo

Calcium is important too, because of its synergistic relationship with magnesium. Although most people associate calcium deficits with poor bone health, low levels can also increase your vulnerability to high blood pressure. But you must be careful about the amount of calcium you take. More than 2,000 mg of calcium per day can cause your kidneys to excrete magnesium!

Chelation Therapy Cleanses Arteries

As discussed earlier, organic calcium is essential for maintaining the health of the brain, heart and nervous system. However, inorganic calcium can be deadly! It can't be absorbed or assimilated by the body and is therefore deposited in joints (arthritis), especially along the artery walls. There it not only hardens arteries and makes them brittle, but also collects deposits of excess cholesterol, forming plaques that clog and impede flow of blood. Chelation Therapy helps remove these plaques.

Within the last fifty years this process known as Chelation Therapy has been carefully developed which removes these abnormal deposits of inorganic calcium from arterial walls and other parts of the body without disturbing the normal balance of organic calcium. Results have been termed "miraculous" by physicians as well as patients. We discuss Chelation Therapy in detail in our book *Healthy Heart.* See back pages for book ordering.

There Are Many Ways to Stop Anxiety & Depression

Depression can be caused by loss, grief, low thyroid, pancreatic cancer, brain trauma, toxins, obesity, diabetes, sleep apnea and more. It is estimated that nearly 30-40% of all depressions have underlying medical causes. If you feel anxious or depressed and it lasts more than two weeks, make sure to get a thorough medical workup,

Alzheimer's Takes Heavy Toll on Women

According to a report from the Alzheimer's Association, Alzheimer's takes a disproportionate toll on women who are far more likely to develop the fatal disease than men. One in six women over 65 will get it during their lifetime, compared with one in 11 men. Alzheimer's is nearly as lethal as heart disease, cancer and breast cancer, because there is no treatment to change the course of the disease. Alzheimer's is currently ranked as the sixth leading cause of death in the U.S. but recent estimates indicate that the disorder may rank third behind heart disease and cancer as a cause of death for older people. Nationwide we'll spend about $214 billion this year on the disease. In fact, Alzheimer's cases are expected to more than triple by 2050! – for more info see www.USAToday.com.

including comprehensive blood work that includes a detailed look at your thyroid. Before trying medication, unless your condition is severe, try some simple healthy interventions such as:

- **Exercise (walk for 45 minutes a day).** In a study comparing exercise to antidepressants, they were equally effective at 12 weeks, and exercise was more effective at 10 months (see more on walking page 112).
- **Eat a healthy, anti-inflammatory diet.** Get rid of the processed foods and sugar, especially foods that quickly turn to sugar. A Mediterranean Diet was shown to have antidepressant effects (see more page 93).
- **Take fish oil to boost Omega-3's**, especially in the form of EPA; start with 3,000 mg of fish oil a day.
- **Work with a therapist** to kill the ANTs (Automatic Negative Thoughts) that fuel depression. Negative thinking patterns can cause anxiety and depression.
- **Check out TMS** (Transcranial Magnetic Stimulation) Treatment (see page 183), which is FDA approved for depression with very few side effects.

For more info see web: *DoctorOz.com*

Take an Active Role in Your Own Health Care

The *Choosing Wisely Initiative* makes patient responsibility in health care a more realistic and practical goal. The Initiative, a joint effort led by American Board of Internal Medicine Foundation and *Consumer Reports*, provides specific medical information to help you make good choices for your medical care. The information comes directly from physician organizations, more than **50 medical specialty societies have submitted more than 200 evidence-based recommendations, including tests and treatments that are often overused, misused or could cause more harm than good.** When a doctor recommends a test or treatment, you can review the *Choosing Wisely* recommendations and discuss them with your doctor. In many situations, consumers are asking for tests and treatments that don't work.

Violence and anger inhibits peace, health and spiritual growth.

Consumer Reports believes that many patients are doing so because of advertisements, promotions, or advice they have received from parts of **the health industry that are too focused on selling something rather than taking care of someone! Surveys have shown that more than 85% of patients had no idea why a particular test was being done, what the risks were, or what the results mean. Some people are harmed by tests that they should never have gotten. The issue isn't cost, it's harm.**

The thought of questioning your doctor is not easy for many people, but you should always discuss tests with your doctors. They should have a good reason to order a test. If you have concerns or need more information to comply with a doctor's orders, it is in your best interest to speak up. Being healthy means being informed about your health. Make a commitment to ask questions at every doctor's visit. If you don't understand something, don't be afraid to speak up. For a complete list of recommendations from the *Choosing Wisely Initiative* go to: *www.ChoosingWisely.org.*

BEWARE OF DEADLY ASPARTAME SUGAR SUBSTITUTES! Although its name sounds "tame," this deadly neurotoxin is anything but! Aspartame is an artificial sweetener (over 200 times sweeter than sugar) made by Monsanto Corporation and marketed as "NutraSweet," "Equal," "Spoonful," and countless other names. Although aspartame is added to over 9,000 food products, it's not fit for human consumption! This toxic poison changes into formaldehyde in the body and has been linked to migraines, seizures, vision loss and symptoms relating to lupus, Parkinson's Disease, Multiple Sclerosis and other health destroying conditions (even Gulf War Syndrome). For more info on this toxic killer – this crime against our health, check web: AspartameKills.com.

A strong, healthy body makes the mind strong.
– Thomas Jefferson, 3rd U.S. President

Progress is impossible without change, and those who cannot change their minds, cannot change anything.
– George Bernard Shaw, 1880's

Cheerfulness is the atmosphere in which all things thrive. – Jean Paul Richter

Relief is on the Way for Nervous Tension, Stress & Anxiety

Here's One of the Main Causes of Nervous Tension, Stress and Anxiety

Amazingly nervous tension, stress and anxiety are caused often by an increased production of hormone-producing glands, including the thyroid, parathyroid, adrenal glands, thymus, hypothalamus, pituitary as well as the ovaries and testes. The hormones of the endocrine glands work to keep the body in a state of normal balance, acting chemically on the body organs to keep growth, appetite, blood pressure, heart rate, sexual drive, and other bodily processes running smoothly. *"Certain glands have more functions than others,"* explains Dr. Mark Gold, author of *The Good News About Panic, Anxiety & Phobias. "The tiny hypothalamus acts as a master gland, regulating all the body's processes, from the sleep/wake cycle to heart rate, hunger and emotions. When it seems unbalanced, it orders the appropriate gland to produce the needed level of the correct hormone to reestablish equilibrium."* Most endocrine problems arise when a particular gland fails to produce the proper amount of hormone. The brain notices the imbalance immediately, and the mind, emotions and behavior can all be affected.

Almost all body functions and organs react to nervous tension, stress and anxiety. The pituitary gland increases its production of adrenal hormones, which in turn stimulates the release of the hormones, cortisone and cortisol. These have the effect of inhibiting the functioning of disease-fighting white blood cells and suppressing the immune response. Increased adrenaline production causes the body to step up its metabolism of protein, fats, and carbohydrates to quickly produce energy for the body to use. This response causes the body to store less calcium, excrete vital amino acids, potassium and phosphorus and depletes magnesium stored in muscle tissue. The body does not absorb ingested nutrients well when under stress, nervous tension or anxiety and therefore becomes deficient in many nutrients. Nervous tension, stress and anxiety also promote the formation of free radicals that can become oxidized and damage body tissues, especially cell membranes. Researchers have found that nearly 80% of all major illnesses, including cardiovascular disease, cancer, endocrine and metabolic diseases, skin disorders, back problems and other physical ailments, are believed to be related to stress, nervous tension and anxiety. **B-complex vitamins are very helpful for proper functioning of the nervous system. Anti-stress enzymes such as L-Tyrosine, as well as calcium, zinc, magnesium, melatonin, SAMe, ginkgo biloba and St. John's Wort are also helpful (see pages 181-182, 185).**

Chronic Depression May Lead to Cancer

According to researchers at the National Institute on Ageing in Bethesda, they tracked 4,825 elderly Americans for 10 years, and found that those who were chronically depressed during the first six years of the study were almost twice as likely to develop cancer as their non-depressed counter-parts. (See web: *Depression.org*) Cancer malignancies of the breast, colon, lung and prostate were prominent in chronically depressed individuals. The researchers stated that depression cannot be considered a cause for cancer, but they noted that depression boosts blood levels of stress hormones, which impair immune function. Chronic depression appears to suppress the immune system significantly enough and long enough to allow cancer cells to multiply.

Link Between Stress and Cancer

According to Scientists at the National Cancer Institute (*Cancer.gov*); psychological stress can affect the immune system, your body's defense against diseases such as cancer. Your body responds to stress by releasing hormones such as adrenalin and cortisol which help you react to a stressful situation by giving you more strength and speed. However, stress hormones increase your blood pressure, heart rate, and blood sugar levels.

Prolonged chronic stress can dangerously increase your risk for obesity; depression; and abuse of drugs and alcohol. Studies also found that chronic stress can affect cancer tumor growth and weaken your immune system.

Importance of Normalizing Blood Pressure

A recent Mayo Clinic study found nearly 40% of the participants who had high blood pressure were unaware of their condition, and only 17% of those with the problem had it under control. Researchers were especially concerned because these participants lived in prosperous communities and had easy access to health care. When left untreated, *this silent killer* – high blood pressure increases a person's risk for heart disease, stroke and kidney failure. Although high blood pressure is predominant in men; after the age of 55 – men and women are at equal risk! Blood pressure is the force of blood against the vessel walls. Systolic pressure is the pressure of the blood in the vessels as the heart beats. Diastolic pressure is the pressure of the blood between heartbeats. If your systolic pressure is 140 or above, and diastolic pressure is 90 or above, it is considered high. Unfortunately, high blood pressure has no symptoms, so it's important to have your blood pressure checked regularly.

To aid in lowering your blood pressure follow these important tips: Lose excess weight; increase physical activity that helps strengthen heart, blood vessels and helps you lose weight. Exercise 30 minutes daily; reduce sodium (salt) in your diet; limit or better yet, stop alcohol – it harms the body, brain, etc. and raises blood pressure, plus adds unnecessary calories. Increase your potassium intake – found in fruits and vegetables. Potassium helps to normalize blood pressure and the body's vital acid/alkaline balance.

CoQ10 for Heart Disease, Cancer, Gum Disease & Ageing

- ***90-120 mgs CoQ10 daily as preventive in cardiovascular & periodontal disease***
- ***120 to 240 mgs CoQ10 daily for angina pectoris, high blood pressure, cardiac arrhythmia and gingivitis (gum disease)***
- ***240-450 mgs daily for congestive heart failure & dilated cardiomyopathy***

– Dr. Stephen T. Sinatra, author of "Coenzyme Q10 Phenomenon"
• healthydirection.com

High blood pressure can lead to decline in some mental abilities, according to researchers at the University of Maine. Elevated blood pressure is a strong predictor of changes in brain structure and related cognitive functioning.

Hypertension Can Be Prevented

According to Scientists, we all carry a salt gene, called angiotensinogen, that can affect our blood pressure. Those with mutated forms of this gene are more likely to develop high blood pressure, say Researchers in the *The Journal of Hypertension*. Blood pressure declines in people with this altered gene when they use less salt. The American Heart Association recommends no more than 2,400 mgs of sodium daily.

Read labels! All cured meats (salami, bacon, hot), frozen dinners, canned foods, soups, chilis and pretzels, chips, and snack foods contain lots of salt. Sweets such as cookies, cakes and soft drinks are loaded with sodium and sugar – best to avoid them! Instead, consume lots of calcium and potassium rich foods; both of these minerals have healthy beneficial effects on blood pressure. For further hypertension info check this website: *MedicineNet.com.*

Combating Depression, Stress & Anxiety

According to the APA – American Psychiatric Association, the good news about depression is that it's more treatable than ever. It's common to get *the blues* when you are disappointed or lose a job or a loved one. However, when diagnosed accurately, there's virtually no one who can't be helped, says Dr. John McIntyre, of the APA. Patients who have used long-term antidepressant prescription drugs found these drugs cause side-effects of drowsiness, insomnia, headaches, nausea and other gastrointestinal symptoms. There are many non-drug therapies available to combat depression that have no side-effects.

"Herbal medicines can be effective in treating anxiety and stress, but they work best when they are part of a natural self-healing program." notes Dr. Harold H. Bloomfield, author of *Healing Anxiety with Herbs*. Kava Herbal Extract is a natural tranquilizer, and as effective as the drug Benzodiazepine Serax (Oxazepam). Kava is a member of the pepper tree family and is used widely in Europe for treating anxiety and insomnia. Other helpful herbs are: St. John's Wort, SAMe, valerian, chamomile,

California poppy, hops, passion flower, ginseng, milk thistle, ginkgo biloba, licorice root, Ashwagandha, Reishi mushrooms and rauwolfia serpentina. Do seek sound health advice and the treatment which will bring you the best health results!

Researchers have shown that those who enjoy a healthy active lifestyle are the most resistant to stress and anxiety! Adopt an active lifestyle that includes 30 minutes or more of daily exercise; stretching your muscles and body to allow a natural open flow of energy; eating healthy nutritional meals; and if possible enjoying a herb and veggie garden. We recommend Bragg follower and licensed nutritionist, Liana Werner-Grey's new book, *Anxiety Free with Food.*

More Stress Relieving Suggestions:

- **Gardening** – researchers have found that to garden helps relieve tensions and is a powerful natural medicine for emotional, spiritual and physical healing.
- **Enjoy natural beauty** – scientific studies indicate that when individuals view beautiful natural scenes such as waterfalls, trees, animals and flowers, they relieve anxiety, relax more easily and feel happier.
- **Reduce or better yet – stop caffeine**, which is a stimulant that can trigger panic attacks and heart palpitations.
- **Stop smoking** – which "burns up" your nervous system.
- **Unplug the phone and computer** – for quiet time can help relieve stress. Write yourself a loving letter.
- **Deep slow breathing exercises** will release tensions.
- **Releasing your fears** and overcoming self-doubt.
- **Restful sleep** and even some daytime mini "cat" naps.
- **Laughter** – people who know how to laugh, smile and have fun are generally able to bounce back from stress.
- **Don't be afraid to ask for help** when you need it!
- **Don't make impulsive snap judgements** – take time.
- **Realize that you can't change the past** – learn from your past pain and let it serve your inner growth.
- **You can't change others** – only change yourself and attitude! Be your strong, positive health captain.

Soothing Remedies for Tension Headaches

Ginger *(Zingiber officinale)* is helpful for tension headaches because it helps decrease production of pain-causing prostaglandins. Also the simple pleasure of taking a break to make and drink a cup of herbal tea will promote a feeling of relaxation and helps to relieve tension and stress. Also try combining ginger with chamomile, peppermint and linden blossom (mild relaxants). Have up to 4 cups daily. Here are the recipes for this ginger-herbal tea and other remedies for soothing tension. Relax and enjoy!

Linden-Flower Tea

To relieve nervous tension and promote relaxation, add 1 tsp of the following herb mixture to 1 cup (8 oz) boiling water:

2 oz linden-flowers
1 oz sage,
1 oz thyme,
1 oz lemon balm.

Steep 15 minutes & strain. Drink 1 hour before bed.

Ginger–Herbal Tea

Simmer 2 tsps fresh grated ginger or powered ginger in 2 cups distilled water in covered pan, 5 minutes. Add:

2 tsps dried linden blossoms
1 tsp each of dried chamomile & peppermint leaves.

Cover & steep for 15 minutes. Then strain & sweeten with honey or herb stevia if desired and enjoy!

Kava Herbal Tea

The Herb Kava, 1/2 tsp of extract tincture in juice, will help relieve tension headaches in five minutes. Also helps relax the muscles in the neck and shoulders and relieves anxiety.

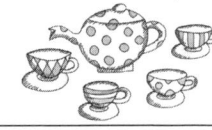

Foods Can Trigger Stress-Related Migraines

Researchers in London reported that after studying 88 children with severe migraines who had eliminated "trigger" foods from their diet, 78 of the children improved greatly. In adults, between 20 to 50% have a reduction of their headaches when trigger foods are avoided! Trigger foods have a reaction in the blood vessels and nerves which causes migraines. The trigger foods to avoid are: dairy products, chocolate, sugars, sodas, eggs and meat.

Headache Acupressure Points

Apply thumb pressure lightly on these pressure points.

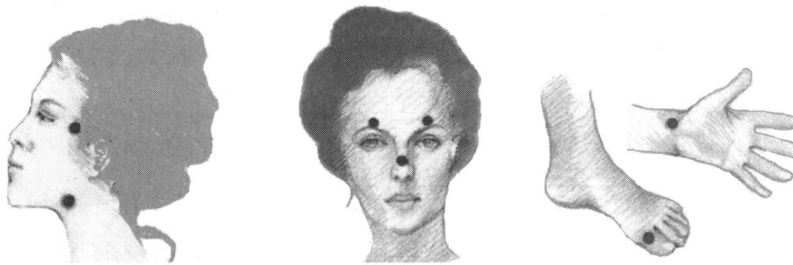

Scientists Reveal Certain Foods Can Alter Moods

If you want to relieve stress naturally you may want to reach for carbohydrate-rich foods such as fresh fruits, vegetables, whole grain breads, cereals and pastas. These elevate serotonin levels which scientists have found help people feel more relaxed and calm. Judith Wurtman, former Director of the Program in Women's Health at Massachusetts Institute of Technology's Brain and Cognitive Sciences Department, and author of *Managing Your Mind and Mood Through Food* says, *"When people consume enough carbohydrates – between 35 to 40 grams – on an empty stomach, they will have the edge taken off their mood and feel better. Low serotonin levels are linked with increased aggression and depression."* Wurtman's research has also shown that high protein foods such as beans, nuts and soy products, release other substances that increase alertness and allow people to react and think more quickly. Studies done revealed that a diet containing omega-3 fat, is responsible for a decreased risk of depression, because it helps manipulate brain chemicals to boost mood. Omega-3 fats can be found in ground flaxseed and walnuts.

SAMe: A Safe Natural Antidepressant

SAMe (S-AdenosylMethionine), is an effective nutritional supplement that helps lift the clouds of depression and fortifies aching joints! According to a health article involving dozens of European trials that involved thousands of patients, SAMe has performed as well as traditional treatments for major depression and arthritis. Research also suggests SAMe can ease normally intractable liver conditions as well. SAMe hasn't shown adverse effects, and doctors have prescribed it successfully for two decades in 14 countries where it has been approved as a drug. SAMe has been successfully used in Europe for over 20 years. SAMe's benefits were first reported in 1973 in Italy, where it is commonly recommended for depression. In one study, researchers found that SAMe worked as well as the prescription antidepressants like Elavil, Norpramin and Prozac without their toxic side effects. **SAMe has been shown to increase levels of happy chemicals in the brain, such as serotonin and dopamine** – without side effects such as agitation, nausea, insomnia and headaches, which are common in prescribed antidepressants (see web: *lef.org*).

In treating osteoarthritis, SAMe has proven beneficial and safe; 71% of a test group had very good results. SAMe was shown to be as effective and even better than Motrin, Advil, Naprosyn and Aleve. Studies also found that SAMe helps restore and maintain damaged cartilage.

SAMe is a naturally occurring molecule found in virtually all body tissues and fluids. It acts as a methyl donor in biochemical reactions and is therefore involved in producing and processing a wide range of chemicals that maintain normal cell function. Since it is a naturally occurring substance, SAMe appears less likely to cause adverse side effects than synthesized drugs. Low levels of SAMe in your blood hinders the liver's efficiency to cleanse toxins from your body. **SAMe supports and promotes the health of many body functions, including joint mobility and comfort, mood and emotional well-being.**

St. John's Wort Relieves Depression

St. John's Wort was named for John the Baptist in the Bible, whose birthday, June 24, falls near the time this plant produces its flowers. The word *wort* means *plant* in Old English. St. John's Wort (*hypericum perforatum*), has been used in traditional herbal medicines for many centuries, primarily for wound healing. Recently, researchers believe this plant is also an SSRI – a class of antidepressant medication. A major study published in the *British Medical Journal,* showed that 55% of the 1,751 patients tested, had depression relief with St. John's Wort. The relief obtained was similar to that experienced from prescription antidepressants. St. John's Wort usually costs about $20 a month, considerably less than pharmaceutical antidepressants, and it does not cause the toxic side effects of other SSRIs. However, St. John's Wort sometimes may cause a dry mouth, some itching and a sensitive stomach. Don't take St. John's Wort when you are taking a pharmaceutical antidepressant (see web: *nccih.nih.gov/health/stjohnswort/sjw-and-depression.htm*)

St. John's Wort contains hypericin with anti-inflammatory properties and was used historically to relieve nerve pain especially resulting from injury, strain and shingles.

Depression & Transcranial Magnetic Stimulation

TMS is a pulsed magnetic field that creates electrical current in the surface of the brain that "resets" the patient's mood regulatory system. You spend just over half an hour in a chair with a powerful magnet affixed to the front left side of your head. TMS is approved specifically for patients whose depression does not respond to antidepressants or cannot tolerate its side effects. Another advantage of TMS treatment is that it is not invasive, and uses no anesthesia or sedation and has few side effects. It does not generally produce seizures and it does not take a toll on memory and cognition, as electroconvulsive therapy can.

Enhance Mood and Mind with Vitamin B1

For decades, researchers have known vitamin B1 *(thiamine – often called the morale vitamin)* has a strong relationship to a healthy nervous system and mental attitude. To test the vitamin's mental status, researchers conducted a study of 120 female college students. The women were split into 2 groups, one taking 50 mg of B1 daily for 2 months and the other receiving a placebo. At study's end, researchers found B1 improved moods and also was safe and effective! Safe dosage of B1 is 50 to 100 mg. (Remember, natural supplements are the best.)

Help For Bipolar Disorder Mood Swings

Fish oil (omega-3) helps calm the volatile mood swings that are the hallmark of bipolar disorder – also known as manic depression. In a 4 month study of 30 people with bipolar disorder (*Prevention.com*), those who took fish oil supplements in addition to their regular medication, saw greater improvement in symptoms than those who did not. Fish oil is rich in omega-3 fatty acids, which seem to tone down the over-active signaling between brain cells that may contribute to mood swings, according to medical researchers at the Baylor College of Medicine in Houston, Texas. See web: *www.bcm.edu*

Very small amounts of vitamin B1 are found in virtually all foods and many commonly eaten foods contain substantial amounts. The best source vitamin B1 is Asparagus. You will also find it in sunflower seeds, navy beans, black beans, barley, dried peas, green peas, lentil, pinto beans, lima beans and oats.

More Natural Remedies for Mood Swings

NADH: the coenzyme in the form of vitamin B3, niacin, helps convert the amino acid tyrosine into the important brain chemical dopamine. Dopamine is involved in mood, energy and sexual drive. According to Austrian researchers, NADH energizes both body and brain activity and improves alertness, concentration, emotions, drive and overall mood enhancement.

Vinpocetine: an Herbal Extract from the periwinkle plant, can dilate blood vessels, enhance circulation to the brain, make red blood cells more pliable, act as an antioxidant and inhibit aggregation of platelets. Researchers have found that vinpocetine appears to be beneficial in cognitive disorders that are due to poor blood flow to the brain. Individuals with atherosclerotic vascular disease may benefit from vinpocetine.

Acetyl-L-Carnitine: helps in energy metabolism and the production of acetylcholine – a brain chemical involved in memory. It can remove toxic accumulations of fatty acids from the mitochondria, keeping these organelles healthy and functioning at their best; helps stabilize cell membranes and protect synapses and brain cells against damage from oxidation. Researchers in Milan, Italy, at the famous Mario Negri Institute for Pharmacological Research, found that acetyl-L-carnitine helped lower the rate of deterioration from Alzheimer's disease and age-related cognitive decline.

Huperzine-A: is an extract from club moss, and has inhibited acetylcholinesterase, the enzyme that breaks down acetylcholine in the brain. Alzheimer's disease is a condition in which there's a relative shortage of acetylcholine. Scientists at Zhejiang Medical University in China, have found that Alzheimer's patients treated with Huperzine-A had improvements in memory and other mental abilities. Other beneficial supplements are: Ginkgo Biloba, SAMe, St. John's Wort (pages 181-182, 185).

Avoid Health-Destroying Habits: Sugar, fat, salt, refined foods and refined flours, chemical preservatives, soda, soft drinks and alcohol.

The greatest mistake you can make in life is to be continually fearing a mistake you might never make. – Elbert Hubbard, 1885

Ginkgo biloba Helps Depression, Stroke and Brain Recovery

Ginkgo biloba improves blood flow through the brain and aids in stroke recovery and mental acuity. It appears to normalize neurotransmitter levels and can help treat depression. In one European study, 80 mg of ginkgo biloba extract was given three times a day to a test group of 40 elderly individuals. After a few months, depression lifted and their mental faculties improved significantly. People taking blood thinners should probably avoid ginkgo until off the blood thinners.

Candida – A Fungus Linked to Chronic Fatigue, Bloating and Nausea

According to Joseph Pizzorno Jr., N.D., author of *Total Wellness*, "Candida (a fungus) in some parts of the body such as the stomach and the vagina, can be relieved by lowering your intake of refined sugars. Sugar is the preferred food of fungi! Even those suffering from ulcers, have higher levels of fungi in their systems." To improve your health and rid yourself of candida it is advised that you dramatically decrease the amount, or better yet, it's best to stop all refined carbohydrates – not only sugar and sweet products, but also white-flour products in your diet. Dr. Pizzorno says you can help combat fungi naturally by taking the following:

Garlic: An anti-fungal agent; use 1 tsp. powder daily, or 1-2 cloves (mashed over salads, veggies, soups, and sauces).

Caprylic Acid: a type of beneficial saturated fatty acid that has antibacterial, antiviral, antifungal and anti-inflammatory properties; use: 1,000 mg tablet with a meal.

Healthy Benefits from Eating Garlic

Ancient Egyptians and Romans prized the extraordinary healing powers of garlic. Garlic has potent immune-enhancing properties. It may eradicate many types of bacteria and fungi, including salmonella and candida, as well as inhibit gastrointestinal ulcers. Garlic's papery skin should be peeled off and the hard roots trimmed at the end. After you chop garlic, let it sit for 10 minutes before cooking or eating, to let the beneficial enzymes develop.

The Fast Growing Healing Revolution: Alternative Health Therapies

According to new millennium studies reported in the *Journal of the American Medical Association*, nearly two-thirds of the nation's 125 traditional U.S. medical schools now teach alternative therapies including: massage, chiropractic, acupuncture, herbal medicine and mind-body medicine. Integrative medicine – a blending of complementary and alternative medicine – is the fastest growing segment of the healthcare industry! A study found 1 in 3 Americans had used alternative therapies, spending over 18 billion annually. This consumer-driven movement is now being joined by physicians who used to scoff at holistic medicine, and by many health insurers who previously had refused to pay for holistic therapies. *"The high-cost and purely scientific approach to medicine needs serious rethinking,"* said Dr. Samuel Benjamin, Director for the National Center for Complementary and Integrative Health, New York's Stony Brook School of Medicine.

"Complementary and Integrative Health is forcing U.S. healthcare to look at different approaches to healthcare, also achieving healthier communities."

The U.S. Congress agrees and has significantly raised its funds appropriated for the National Center for Complementary and Alternative Medicine, upwards of $150 million in 2020 This is a positive step towards better health for Americans!

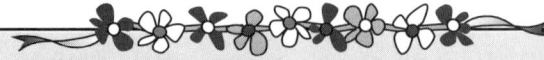

Oil Pulling May Transform Your Health

The ancient Ayurvedic remedy for oral health and detoxification is in oil pulling. It involves the use of pure oils such as organic sesame, coconut or olive oil, as agents for pulling harmful bacteria, fungus and other organisms out of the mouth, teeth, gums and even the throat. All you need to do is place about a tablespoon of oil into your mouth and swish it around for approximately 10-15 minutes, then spit it out. Lipids in the oil pulls out toxins from the saliva; the oil absorbs toxins and bacteria. The oil may help in cellular restructuring and proper functioning of the lymph nodes and other internal organs.

Healthy Alternative Therapies and Massage Techniques

Try Them – They Are Working Miracles!

Explore these wonderful natural methods of healing your body. Finally over 600 Medical Schools in the U.S. are teaching Healthy Alternative Therapies. Please check their websites. Now seek and choose the best healing techniques for you:

ACUPUNCTURE / ACUPRESSURE: Acupuncture directs and rechannels body energy by inserting hair-thin needles (use only disposable needles) at specific points on the body. It's used for pain, backaches, migraines and general health and body dysfunctions. Used in Asia for centuries, acupuncture is safe, virtually painless and has no side effects! Acupressure is based on the same principles and uses finger pressure and massage rather than needles. Check web: *AcupunctureToday.com*

CHIROPRACTIC: was founded in Davenport, Iowa in 1885 by Daniel David Palmer. There are now many schools in the U.S., and graduates are joining Health Practitioners in all nations of the world to share healing techniques. Chiropractic is popular and the largest U.S. healing profession benefitting literally millions! Treatment involves soft tissue, spinal and body adjustment to free your nervous system of any interferences with normal body functions. Its concern is the functional integrity of the musculoskeletal system. In addition to manual methods, chiropractors use physical therapy modalities, exercise, health and nutritional guidance. Web: *ChiroWeb.com*

COLON HYDROTHERAPY: is a safe and effective practice for supporting detoxification, and improving health and vitality. Contact I-ACT (Int'l Association Colon Hydrotherapy) for a certified colon Hydro-Therapist in your area. Web: *i-act.org*

SKIN BRUSHING: daily is wonderful for circulation, toning, cleansing and healing. Use a dry vegetable brush (never nylon) and brush lightly. Helps purify lymph so it's able to detoxify your blood and tissues. Removes old skin cells, uric acid crystals and toxic wastes that come up through skin's pores. Use loofah sponge for variety in shower or tub.

Skin is often called the 3rd kidney because it eliminates toxins from body.

HOMEOPATHY: In 1796, Dr. Samuel Hahnemann, a German physician, developed homeopathy. Patients are treated with "micro" doses of remedies found in nature to trigger the body's own defenses. This homeopathic principle is a safe and nontoxic remedy and is the #1 alternative therapy in Europe and Britain because it is inexpensive, seldom has any side effects, and usually brings fast results. Web: *HomeopathyCenter.org*

NATUROPATHY: Brought to America by Dr. Benedict Lust, M.D., this treatment uses diet, herbs, homeopathy, fasting, exercise, hydrotherapy, manipulation and sunlight. Practitioners work with your body to restore health naturally. They reject surgery and drugs except as a last resort. Web: *www.Naturopathic.org*

OSTEOPATHY: The first School of Osteopathy was founded in 1892 by Dr. Andrew Taylor Still, M.D. There are now 30 U.S. colleges. Treatment involves soft tissue, spinal and body adjustments that free the nervous system from interferences that can cause illness. Healing by adjustment also includes good nutrition, physical therapies, proper breathing and good posture. Dr. Still's premise: if the body structure is altered or abnormal, then proper body function is altered and can cause pain and illness. Web: *www.AcademyofOsteopathy.org*

REFLEXOLOGY/ZONE THERAPY: Founded by Eunice Ingham, author of *Stories The Feet Can Tell*, inspired by a Bragg Health Crusade when she was 17. Reflexology helps the body and organs by removing crystalline deposits from reflex areas (nerve endings) of feet and hands through deep pressure massage. Primitive reflexology originated in China and Egypt and Native American Indians and Kenyans self-practiced it for centuries. Reflexology activates your body's flow of healing and energy by dislodging deposits. Visit Eunice Ingham and nephew Dwight Byer's website: *www.Reflexology-usa.net*

WATER THERAPY: Soothing detox shower: apply organic olive oil to skin, alternate hot and cold water, every 2-3 minutes. Massage body while under hot, filtered spray. Garden hose massage is great in summer or anytime. Hot detox soak bath (diabetics use warm water) 20 minutes with cup of Epsom salts or apple cider vinegar. This soak helps pull out the toxins by creating an artificial fever cleanse.

My father and I want you to enjoy a fulfilled, healthy, long life.
– Patricia Bragg, Pioneer Health Crusader

Time waits for no one, treasure and protect every moment you have!

ALEXANDER TECHNIQUE: helps end improper use of neuromuscular system, helps bring body posture into balance. Eliminates psycho-physical interferences, helps release long-held tension, and aids in re-establishing muscle tone. For more info see web: *AlexanderTechnique.com*

FELDENKRAIS METHOD: Dr. Moshe Feldenkrais founded this in the late 1940s. This Method leads to improved posture and helps create ease and more efficiency of body movement. This Method is a great stress removal. Web: *Feldenkrais.com*

REIKI: A Japanese form of massage that means "Universal Life Energy." Reiki Massage helps the body to detoxify, then re-balance and heal itself. Discovered in the ancient Sutra manuscripts by Dr. Mikao Usui in Japan 1922. Web: *Reiki.org*

ROLFING: Developed by Ida Rolf in the 1930's in the U.S. Rolfing is also called structural processing and postural release, or structural dynamics. It is based on the concept that distortions (accidents, injuries, falls, etc.) and the effects of gravity on the body cause upsets and long-term stress in the body. Rolfing helps to achieve balance and improved body posture. Methods involve the use of stretching, with gentle deep tissue massage and relaxation techniques to loosen old injuries, break bad movement and posture patterns. Web: *Rolf.org*

TRAGERING: Founded by Dr. Milton Trager M.D., who was inspired at age 18 by Paul C. Bragg to become a doctor. It is a mind-body learning method that involves gentle shaking and rocking, allowing the body to let go, releasing tensions and lengthening the muscles for more body peace and health. Tragering can do miracle healing where needed in the body frame, muscles and the entire body. Web: *Trager.com*

MASSAGE & AROMATHERAPY: works two ways: the essence (aroma) relaxes, as does healing massages. Essential oils are extracted from flowers, leaves, roots, seeds and barks. These are usually massaged into skin, inhaled or used in a bath to help the body relax, soothe and heal. The oils, used for centuries to treat numerous ailments, are revitalizing and energizing for the body and mind. Example: Tiger balm, MSM, echinacea and arnica help relieve muscle aches. (Avoid skin creams and lotions with mineral oil – it clogs the skin's pores.) Use these natural oils for the skin: almond, avocado, and I use organic olive oil and mix with aromatic essential oils: rosemary, lavender, rose, jasmine, sandalwood or lemon-balm, etc. – 6 oz. oil and 4 drops of an essential oil. Web: *www.Aromatherapy.com*

MASSAGE – SELF: Paul C. Bragg often said, *"You can be your own best massage therapist, even if you have only one good hand."* Near-miraculous health improvements have been achieved by victims of accidents or strokes in bringing life back to afflicted parts of their own bodies by self-massage and with vibrators. Treatments can be day or night, almost continual. Self-massage also helps achieve relaxation at day's end. Families and friends can learn and exchange massages; it's a wonderful sharing experience. Remember, babies love and thrive with daily massages, start from birth. Family pets also love soothing, healing touch of massages. Web: *RD.com/health/wellness/learn-the-art-of-self-massage*

MASSAGE – SHIATSU: Japanese massage form applies pressure from fingers, hands, elbows and even knees along the same points as acupuncture. Shiatsu originated in Japan and is based on traditional Chinese medicine, and has been widely practiced around the world since 1970s. Shiatsu has been used in Asia for centuries to relieve pain, common ills, muscle stress and to aid lymphatic circulation. See web: *centerpointmn.com/the-benefits-of-shiatsu-massage*

MASSAGE – SWEDISH: One of the oldest and the most popular and widely used massage techniques. This deep body massage soothes and promotes healthy circulation and is a great way to loosen and relax tight muscles before and after exercise. See web: *www.MassageDen.com/swedish-massage.shtml*

MASSAGE – SPORTS: An important health support system for professional and amateur athletes. Sports massage improves circulation and mobility to injured tissue, enables athletes to recover more rapidly from myofascial injury, reduces muscle soreness and chronic strain patterns. Soft tissues are freed of trigger points and adhesions, thus contributing to improvement of peak neuromuscular functioning and athletic performance.

Author's Comment: We have personally sampled many of these Alternative Therapies. It's estimated America's health care costs are over $2.6 trillion. It's more important than ever to be responsible for our own health! This includes seeking dedicated holistic health practitioners to keep us well by inspiring us to practice prevention! These Alternative Healing Therapies are also popular and getting results: aromatherapy, Ayurvedic, biofeedback, guided imagery, herbs, hyperbaric oxygen, music, meditation, magnets, saunas, tai chi, Qi gong, Pilates, Rebounder, yoga, etc. Explore them and be open to improving your earthly temple for a healthy, happier, longer life.

Seek and find the best for your body, mind and soul. – Patricia Bragg

Control & Extend Your Health & Lifespan!

In the final analysis, it's up to you! No one can control your eating and living habits except yourself. You may take your troubles to experts, but all they can do is tell you what you should do. They can't do it for you. Most of your problems of living cannot be solved by someone else . . . only you! In this book we have given you the results of a lifetime of experience in the field of natural living and building a Powerful Nerve Force. This is all we can do! Now it's up to you to apply these teachings in your own life, to help solve your own problems and fill your own needs! Our prayers and love go with you daily as you strive to become more peaceful and healthy.

Earn Your Bragging Rights
Live The Bragg Healthy Lifestyle To Attain Supreme Physical, Mental, Emotional and Spiritual Health!

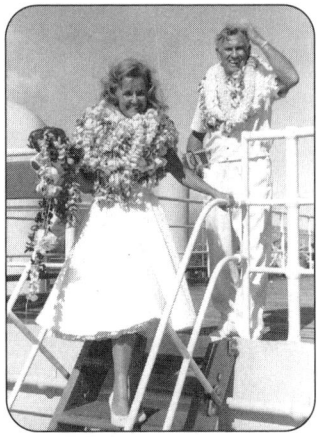

Health Crusaders Paul C. Bragg and daughter Patricia traveled the world spreading health, inspiring millions to renew and revitalize their health.

We have love for you and God loves you – pass it along and share this wisdom and love,

Paul C. Bragg and Patricia Bragg

Genesis 6:3 ***3 John 2***

FROM THE AUTHORS

This book was written for You! It can be your passport to a healthy, long, vital life. We in the Alternative Health Therapies join hands in one common objective – promoting a high standard of health for everyone. Healthy Nutrition points the way – which is Mother Nature and God's Way. This book teaches you how to work with them, not against them! Health Doctors, Therapists, Nurses, Teachers and Caregivers are becoming more dedicated than ever before to keeping their patients healthy and fit. This book was written to emphasize great needed importance of healthy lifestyle living for health and longevity, close to Mother Nature and God.

Statements in this book are scientific health findings, known facts of physiology and biological therapeutics. Paul C. Bragg practiced natural methods of living for over 80 years with highly beneficial results, knowing they were safe and of great value. His daughter Patricia lectured and co-authored Bragg Health Books with him and continues carrying on The Bragg Healthy Lifestyle.

Paul C. Bragg and daughter Patricia express their opinions solely as Public Health Educators and Health Crusaders. They offer no cure for disease. Only the body has the ability to cure a person. Experts may disagree with some of the statements made in this book. However, such statements are considered to be factual, based on the long-time experience of dedicated pioneer Health Crusaders Paul C. Bragg and Patricia Bragg. If you suspect you have a medical problem, please always seek qualified Health Care professionals to help you make the healthiest, wisest and best-informed choices!

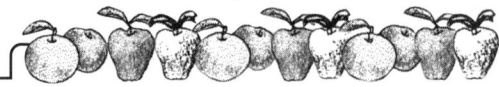

Count your blessings daily while you do your 30 to 45 minute brisk walks and exercises with these affirmations – health! strength! youth! vitality! peace! laughter! humility! understanding! forgiveness! joy! and love for eternity! and soon all these qualities will come flooding and bouncing into your life. With blessings of super health, peace and love to you, our dear friends – our readers. – Patricia Bragg, Health Crusader

If I were to name the three most precious resources of life, I would say books, friends and nature; and the greatest of these, at least the most constant and always at hand is Mother Nature and God. – John Burroughs

Change your lifestyle to healthy living, then you will improve your life!

Everything in excess is opposed by nature. – Hippocrates, Father of Medicine

Praises and Testimonials for The Bragg Healthy Lifestyle

I would like to thank you and your father for inspiring me to live a healthy life. Out of all the health books in the world, I consider yours my health bible. It is the only thing that has rang true to me without question. Thank you for making a difference in my life. – Jo Ann

---

Thank you for your voice trying to protect the public from our pitiful system that is killing us with chemicals. People are too busy with pleasures to be interested in their own health and their precious life! Thanks so much.
– Charles & Elizabeth Belote, Nevada

The Lord works sometimes in ways we don't expect. He chose to answer my prayer by leading me to your health books and way of living . . . thus my medical problems are GONE! I want to give thanks to God, and to you, Patricia and your father. It was the Bragg Health Books that converted me to Healthy Living . . . and I will never be the same again! Thank You and God Bless. – Jimmy Damianos, Florida

---

In the past our family has had chronic health problems. Within the last year and a half God has shown us His Will for healing and divine health. Our journey has included a healthy diet, some fasting and a complete change in lifestyle. I cannot express how good we feel! I am so thankful for every good thing that God has put before us – this journey, and every miraculous result and ACV is part of that. Thank you for sharing this wealth of health in Bragg Books. God Bless You! – Rhonda Jackson, Oklahoma

"You change your life by changing your heart." – Max Lucado

Count your blessings, name them one by one;
count your many blessings, see what God hath done.
– Johnson Oatman, Jr., songwriter
I give thanks for all the Miracle Blessings I receive daily.
– Patricia Bragg

Praises and Testimonials for The Bragg Healthy Lifestyle

I am truly grateful to you. I am going to try my hardest to get my health back and I believe I can do that if I faithfully follow the advise given in your books. Please believe me when I say, the world is a better place due to the gift of you. You truly have a special heart and soul. Thank You and God Bless You. – Bob Evanson

---

Rock and roll health is better than rock and roll wealth. Thanks to Bragg, the road ain't a drag anymore! We thank Bragg for the super smooth going and success on our recent successful whirlwind 20 city tour of England. – David Polemeni, Boy's Town Band, New Jersey

---

Paul Bragg inspired me many years ago with the "Miracle of Fasting" and with his philosophy on health. His daughter Patricia is a testament to the ageless value of living the Bragg Healthy Lifestyle. – Jay Robb, Author, *The Fruit Flush*

The results with Bragg Healthy Lifestyle are miraculous! I got rid of a constant cold and mucus. I feel so good, energetic and healthy again. Thank You! – Nestor R. Villagra, Toronto, Ontario, Canada

Health Habits to Follow

Good health! Whenever you go out of doors, draw the chin in, carry the crown of your head high, and fill the lungs to the utmost; drink in sunshine; greet your friends with a smile, and put soul into every handclasp. Do not fear being misunderstood and never waste a minute thinking about your enemies.

– Elbert Hubbard, American writer, publisher, artist, and philosopher.

The more natural food you eat, the more you'll enjoy radiant health and be able to promote the higher life of love and brotherhood. – Patricia Bragg

---

This is our goal for you – Radiant, Super Health! – 3 John 2

Praises and Testimonials for The Bragg Healthy Lifestyle

The Bragg Healthy Lifestyle, vinegar drink and brisk walking (3x daily) 20 minutes after meals, helped eliminate my diabetes! My whole body, circulation, feet, eyes have all improved. Thank you, may God continue to bless your Bragg Crusade.
– John Risk, CA

I was diagnosed with diabetes and had high sugar levels. Within only 6 months, I was insulin free! I am healthier now than I have been for the past 15 years. My wife, three young children and I are now all healthy vegetarians and living the Bragg Healthy Lifestyle. The results have been amazing!
We all thank You. – Dennis Urbans, Australia

Your general health approach to solving common infirmities is superior to trying to target them. General health is a joy and side effects from Bragg Healthy Lifestyle are none existent. Thank you for the health common sense teachings I have learned from your books.
– John Kalagher, Massachusetts

Thank you for your wealth of health information in the Bragg Books. I have followed a vegetarian diet and your lifestyle for 31 years. It works! I teach school and lifeguard for the Kentucky Department of Parks in the summer. I still swim a mile a day! Thank you and may God continue to bless your health outreach! – Steve House, Kentucky

Do not go where the path may lead. Go instead where there is no path, and thus leave a trail. – Emerson

---

Let your inner light happily shine brightly. – Beatrex Quntanna

---

Change your thoughts and you change your world. – Norman Vincent Peale

Praises and Testimonials for The Bragg Healthy Lifestyle

Thanks for all that you and your father have done for humanity. Those that have listened have benefitted beyond belief. God Bless.
– Terry Sonnenschein, CA

I am truly thrilled by what I've read. I am excited and confident of my now newer ways to keep super healthy.
– Ken Cooper, D.C., Narrabi, NSW, Australia

Thank you for the wonderful knowledge you provide on health. Your books are truly inspirational. I have been following your Healthy Lifestyle for about four months. The way I feel is incredible. I have more energy, a calmer outlook on life and was not aware of all the food choices. I now enjoy all organic fruits and vegetables.
– Maria Poppe, New York

I am following the Bragg Healthy Lifestyle which I heard of through a friend. Your books are motivators and have blessed my health and life and are making perfect gifts for my family and friends. – Delphine, Singapore

---

I have just recently embraced the live food diet and I am overwhelmed at the beauty and simplicity of it all. When we become aligned with Natural Laws the Universe opens up for you and nature does reveal it's mysteries to you!
– Patrick McLean, KS

Good health, generated by physical fitness is the logical starting point for the pursuit of excellence in any field. Physical vitality promotes mental vitality and thus is essential to executive achievement.
– Dr. Richard E, Dutton, University of Southern Florida

Please observe and respect the Laws of Mother Nature and God.

 What sunshine is to flowers, smiles are to humanity. – Joseph Addison

BRAGG PHOTO GALLERY

PATRICIA & PAUL C. BRAGG, N.D., Ph.D.

Dynamic Daughter & Father are World Health Crusaders

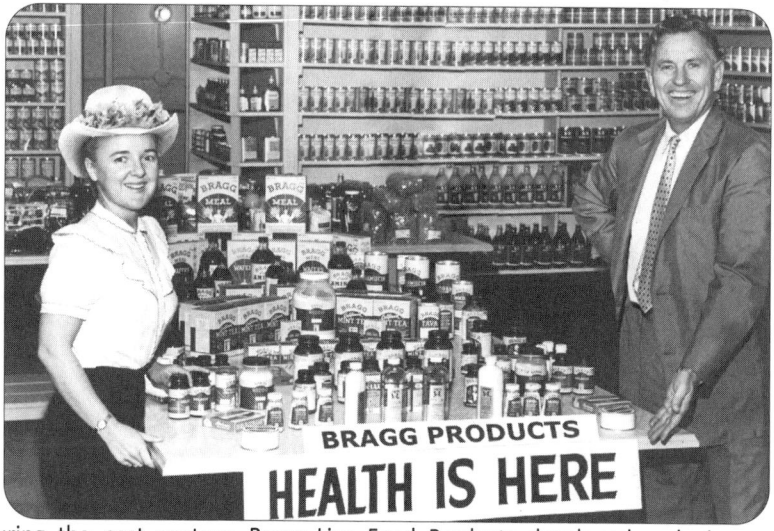

During the past century, Bragg Live Food Products developed and pioneered the very first line of Health Foods, from vitamins and minerals to organic nuts, seeds, and sun-dried fruits. This included over 365 health products, – *"one for each day of the year!"* says daughter Patricia Bragg.

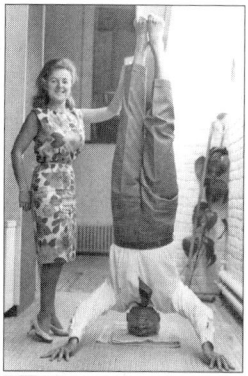

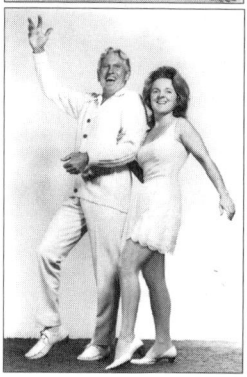

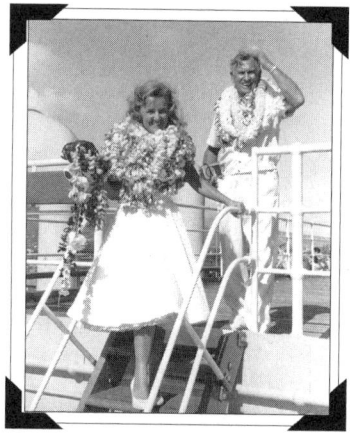

Patricia and father, Paul on world trip in 1950's, during stop in Tahiti.

"You have recharged me with joy, hope, love and encouragement, which poured from your words. I am now fasting and using ACV. You have certainly improved my life!"
– Marie Furia, New Jersey

"Thanks for The Bragg Healthy Lifestyle that you shared with me and you are sharing with millions of others worldwide."
– John Gray, Ph.D., author

Picture from *People Magazine* August, 1975.

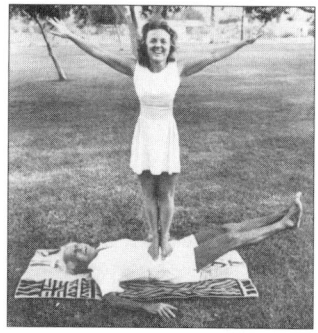

Patricia Bragg stands on her father's stomach. Paul's stomach muscles are so strong he can lift Patricia up and down!

PHOTO GALLERY

PAUL C. BRAGG, N.D., Ph.D.
HEALTH CRUSADER

Life Extension Specialist and Originator of Health Food Stores

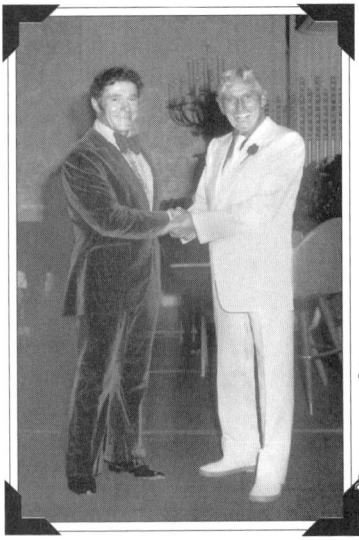

Dr. Paul C. Bragg (right) Creator Health Food Stores, Pioneer Life Extension Specialist, with his prize student Jack LaLanne. Paul started him on the royal road to health over 85 years ago!

I have experienced a beautiful, remarkable, spiritual and physical awakening since reading Bragg Health Books. I'll never be the same again.
– Sandy Tuttle, Ohio

With every new day comes new strength and new thoughts.
– Eleanor Roosevelt

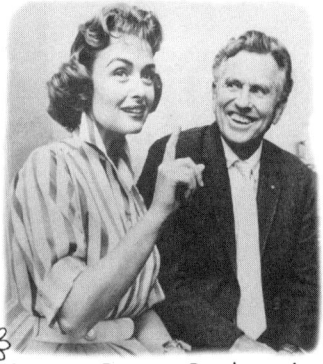

Actress Donna Reed saying "Health First" with Paul C. Bragg.

Paul C. Bragg spent much of his time at the Hollywood Studios meeting with top Stars and motion picture industry executives, giving health lectures and private consultations. Dr. Paul C. Bragg was Hollywood's first highly respected, health, fitness and nutrition advisor to the Stars.

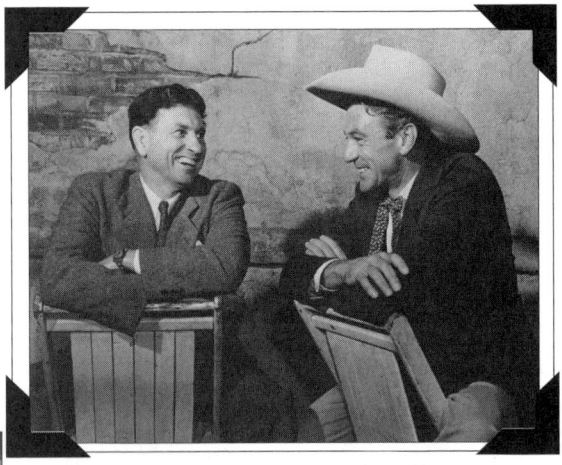

Paul C. Bragg with Gary Cooper, famous American film actor, best known for his many Western films.

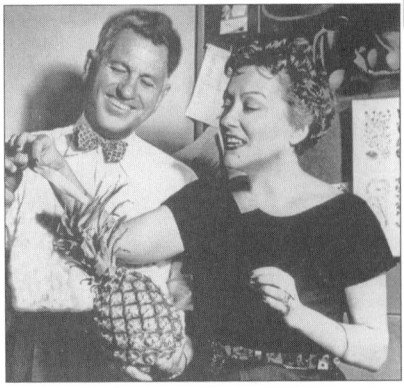

Paul C. Bragg with the famous Hollywood Actress Gloria Swanson, who was leading star in 20s, 30s and 40s. Gloria became a Bragg Health Devotee at 18 and she often would Health Crusade with Bragg during the 1950s.

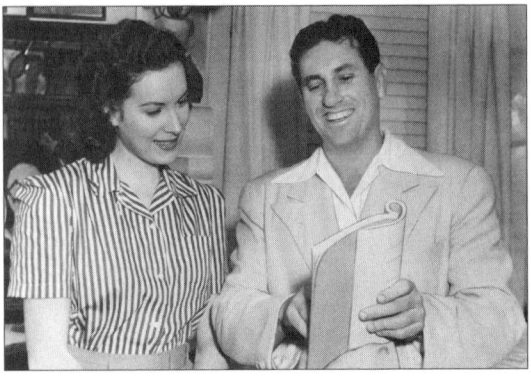

Maureen O'Hara and Paul C. Bragg. This Irish film actress and singer was best noted for playing in "Miracle on 34th Street" and "The Quiet Man."

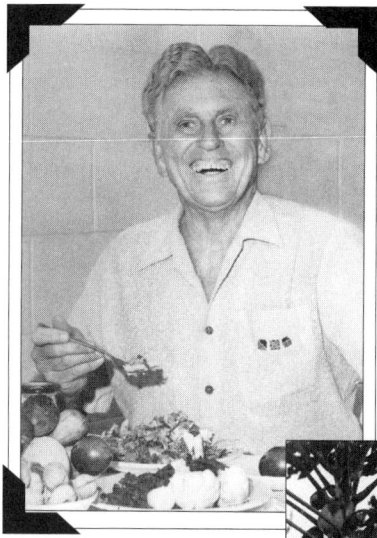

Dr. Paul C. Bragg and daughter Patricia were my early guiding inspiration to my health career.
– Jeffery Bland, Ph.D., Famous Food Scientist

I'd like to thank you for teaching me how to take control of my health! I lost 55 pounds and I feel "great!" Bragg books have showed me vitality, happiness and being close to Mother Nature. You both are real "Crusaders for Health for the World." Thanks!
– Leonard Amato

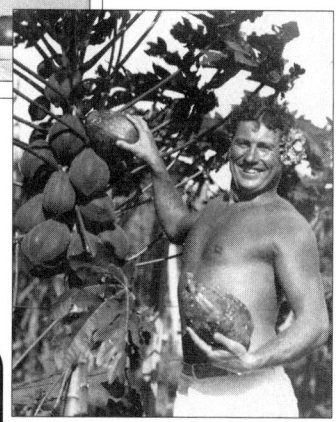

Paul C. Bragg in Tahiti 1920's gathering tropical papaya fruit.

The best thing about the future is that it only comes one day at a time.
– Abraham Lincoln

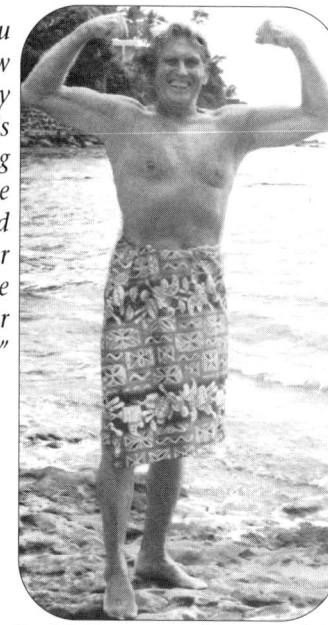

Paul C. Bragg owes his powerful body and superb health to living exclusively on live, vital, healthy, organic rich foods.

Dear Friends – you cannot know how greatly you have impacted my life and some of my friends! We love your Bragg Health Books, teachings and products and are now living healthier, happier lives. Thanks!
– Winnie Brown, Arizona

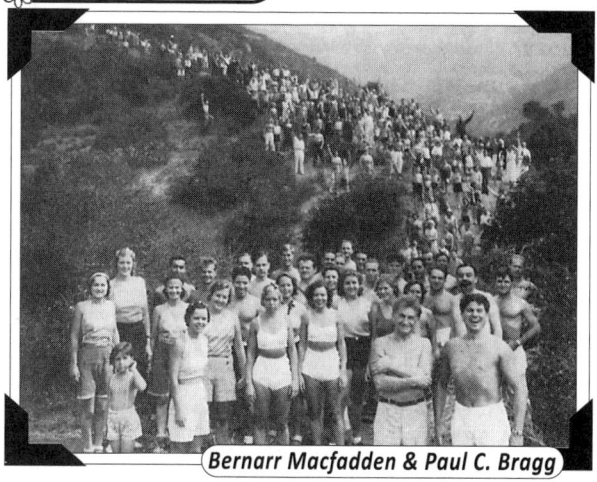

Bernarr Macfadden & Paul C. Bragg

A thousand happy Bragg Health Students enjoy hiking, exercise and fresh air on the trail to Mount Hollywood (above Griffith Observatory) in beautiful California, summer of 1932.

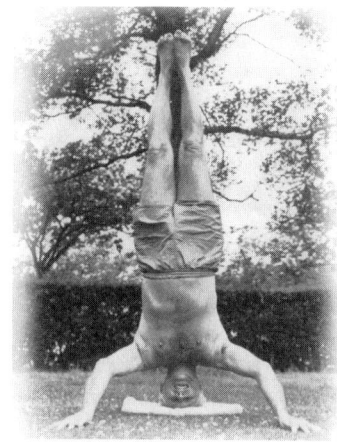

Paul C. Bragg exercising Regent's Park, London.

PHOTO GALLERY PAUL & PATRICIA BRAGG

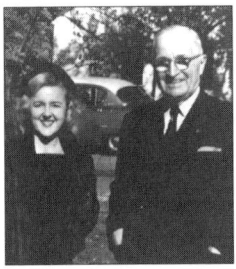

Patricia with 33rd President Harry S. Truman at his home in Independence, Missouri.

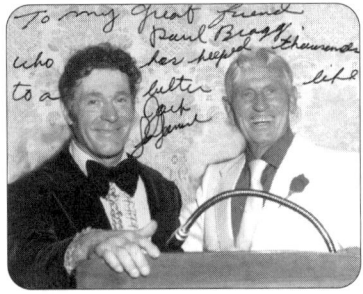

Paul C. Bragg, Creator of Health Food Stores, with his prize student Jack LaLanne, who thanks Bragg for saving his life at 15.

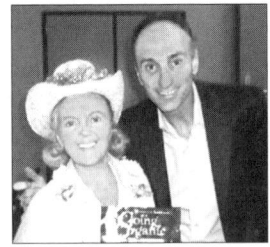

Patrica Bragg with Dr. Jeffrey Smith. He is leader in getting GMO's out of US foods. See GMO video by Jeffrey Smith and narrated by Lisa Oz (Dr. Oz's wife) on web: *GeneticRouletteMovie.com*

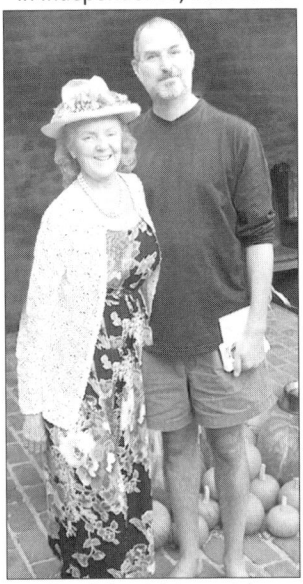

Patricia visiting with Steve Jobs at his home in Palo Alto during the Thanksgiving Holidays.

"I've been reading Bragg Books since high school. I'm thankful for the Bragg Healthy Lifestyle and admire their Health Crusading for a healthier, happier world."
– Steve Jobs, Creator – Apple Computer

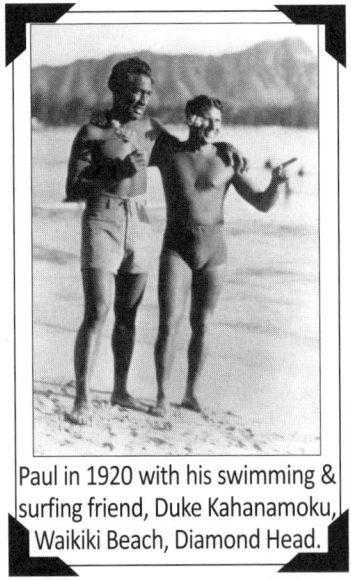

Paul in 1920 with his swimming & surfing friend, Duke Kahanamoku, Waikiki Beach, Diamond Head.

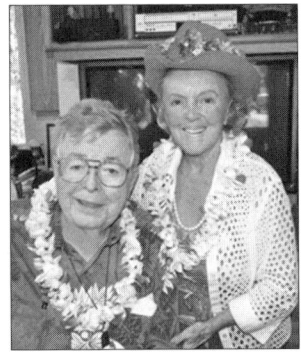

Dr. Earl Bakken with Patricia. He's famous for inventing the first Transistor Pacemaker. His firm Medtronic, developed it and a Resuscitator for fixing ailing hearts that have and are saving thousands of lives. Dr. Bakken lived in Hawaii.

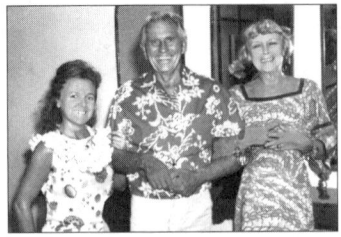

Patricia, Paul C. Bragg and Mrs. Duke (Nadine) Kahanamoku. (Nadine is Patricia's Godmother).

"I cannot remember a time when the Golden Rule was not my motto and precept, the torch that guided my footsteps."* – J.C. Penney

***The Golden Rule:** Do unto others as you would have them do unto you.

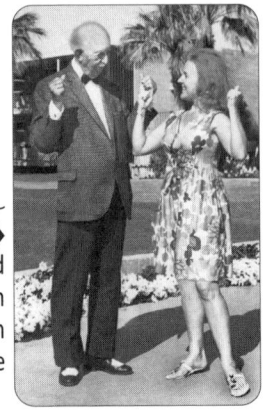

J.C.Penney & Patricia → exercising. They walked often in Palm Springs when he and his wife visited in the winter to enjoy the warm desert sunshine.

HEALTH CRUSADING TO HOLLYWOOD STARS

PHOTO GALLERY

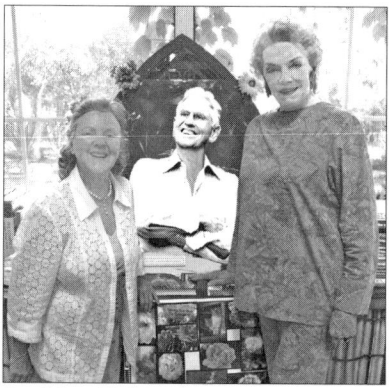

Patricia with friend Actress Jane Russell. Famous Hollywood Star of 40s to 60s.

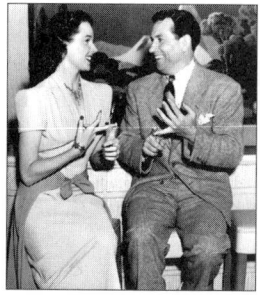

Jane Wyatt learning about health with Paul C. Bragg.

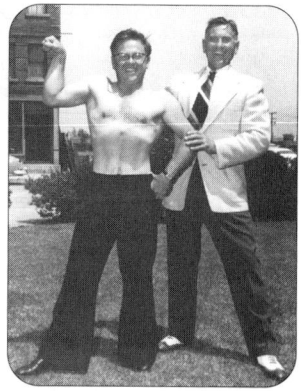

Mickey Rooney with Paul. Rooney was an American film actor and entertainer. He won multiple awards and had one of the longest careers of any actor to age 93!

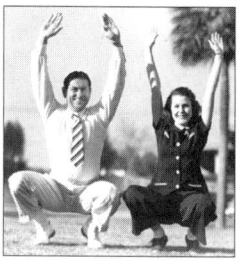

Paul C. Bragg exercising with Actress Helen Parrish.

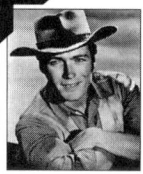

"Thank you Paul & Patricia Bragg for my simple, easy-to-follow Healthy Lifestyle. You make my days healthy!" – Clint Eastwood, Academy Award Winning Film Producer, Director, Actor and Bragg follower for over 65 years.

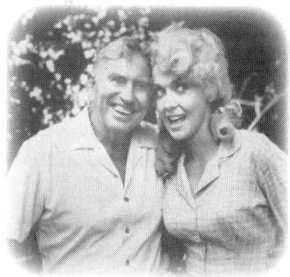

Paul C. Bragg and Donna Douglas, one of Hollywood's most beautiful and talented health advocates. She played the part of "Elly-May" in the *Beverly Hillbillies*, which became one of the longest-running series in television history and was the #1 show in America in its first 2 years.

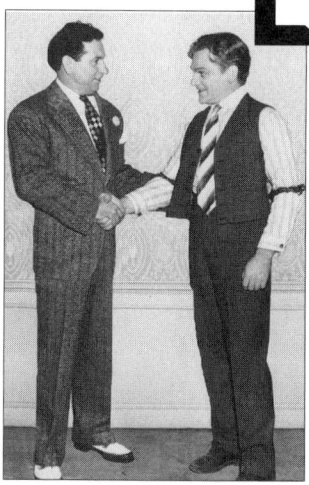

Paul C. Bragg with James Cagney, American film actor. He won major awards for wide variety of roles. The American Film Institute ranked Cagney 8th among the Greatest Male Hollywood Stars of All Time.

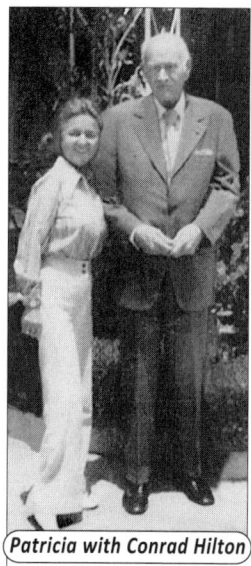

Patricia with Conrad Hilton

Life is a Miracle Minute by Minute Year by Year!

← Hotel founder, Conrad Hilton with Patricia Bragg, his Healthy Lifestyle Teacher. *"I wouldn't be alive today if it wasn't for the Braggs and their Bragg Healthy Lifestyle!"* – Conrad Hilton

"Thank you for your website. What a wealth of info to learn about how to live and eat healthy. Many Blessings!" – Michel & Mary, California

PAUL C. BRAGG, N.D., Ph.D. PROMOTES HEALTH & FITNESS!

Paul C. Bragg leading an exercise class in Griffith Park, Hollywood, CA – circa 1920s.

Bragg Healthy Lifestyle works Miracles! – Jack LaLanne

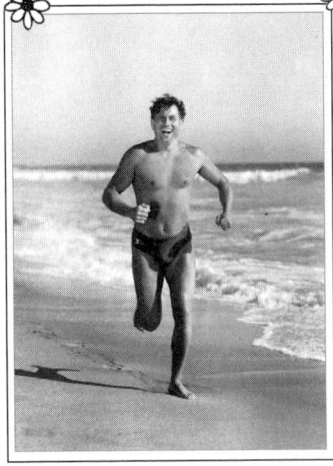

Paul running on Coney Island, New York, where he was a member of the Coney Island Polar Bear Club, known for Cold Water Swimming, 1930s.

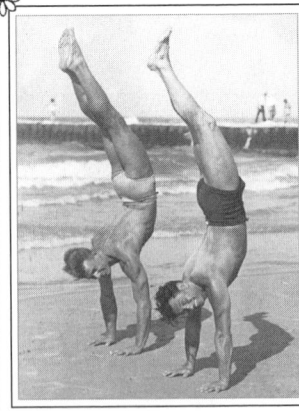

Friend and Paul C. Bragg doing handstand at the beach.

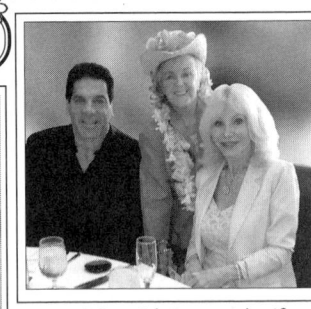

Patricia with Lou and wife Carla at Elaine LaLanne's 90th Birthday Party.

TV Hulk Actor Lou Ferrigno gives thanks to Bragg Books. Lou went from puny to become Super Hulk!

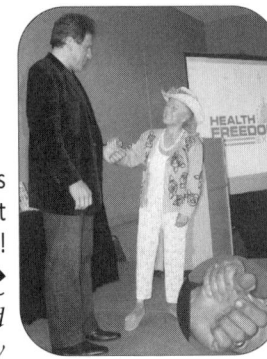

Lou & Patricia in Chicago Health Freedom Expo.

"I lost 102 lbs. with The Bragg Healthy Lifestyle and I have kept it off for over 15 years, staying away from white flour, sugar and other processed foods."
– Dee McCaffrey, Chemist & Diet Counselor, Tempe, AZ

PATRICIA CONTINUING BRAGG HEALTH CRUSADE!

PHOTO GALLERY

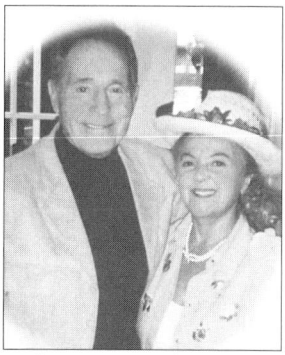

Jack LaLanne with Patricia.

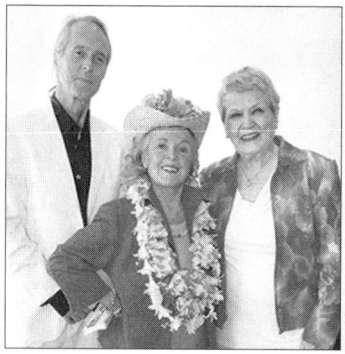

Jon & Elaine LaLanne with Patricia.

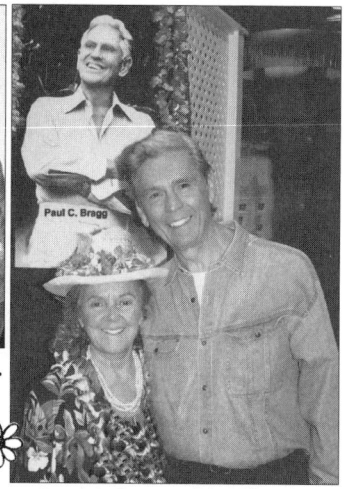

Patricia Bragg with Bill Galt inspired by Bragg Books, he founded Good Earth Restaurants.

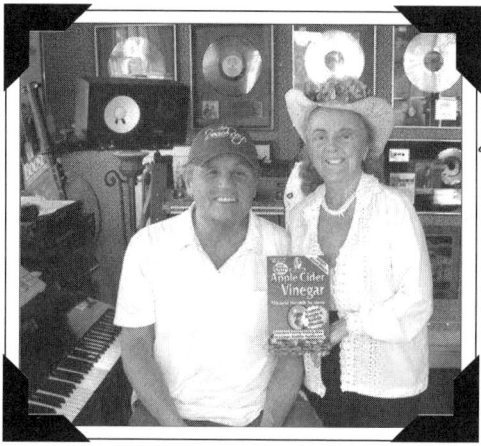

Patricia in studio with famous Beach Boy Bruce Johnston, Bragg follower over 40 years. He played for her their latest records.

Mother Nature Loves US!

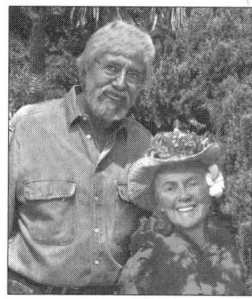

Patricia with Jean-Michel Cousteau Ocean Explorer & Environmentalist. OceanFutures.org

Enjoy a Lifetime of Radiant Health

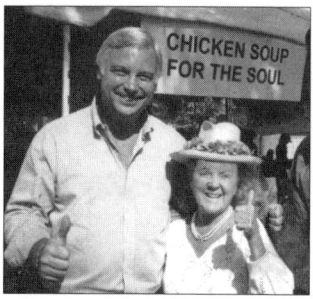

Patricia with Jack Canfield, Bragg follower, Motivational Speaker and Co-Producer of *Chicken Soup For The Soul.*

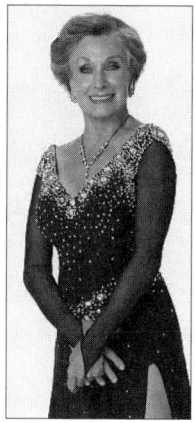

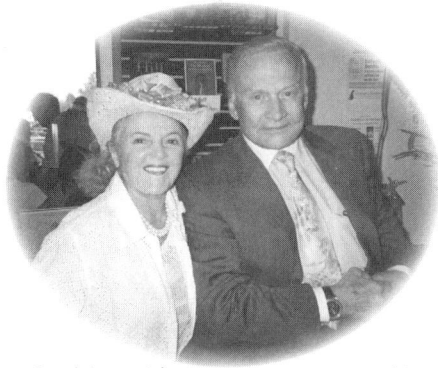

Patricia with Astronaut Buzz Aldrin, celebrating over 50 years since pilot of Apollo 11 first landed on the moon.

Famous Hollywood Actress Cloris Leachman, ardent health follower who sparkled with health and vitality said, *"The Miracle of Fasting Book is a miracle . . . it cured my asthma, my years of arthritis and many other health problems. I praise Paul and Patricia daily for their Health Crusading!"*

PHOTO GALLERY

PAUL & PATRICIA BRAGG HEALTH CRUSADING

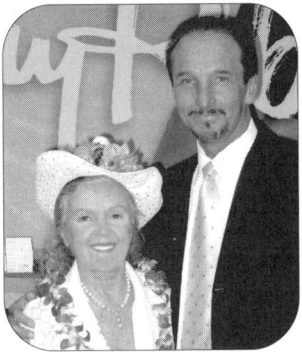

Patricia with Jay Robb.

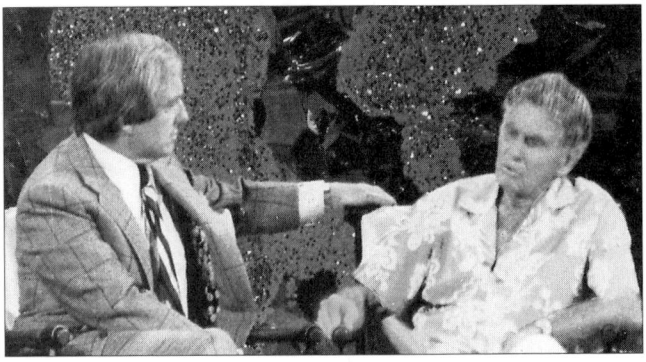

Paul C. Bragg on the Merv Griffin Show, 1976.

Paul Bragg inspired me many years ago with The Miracle of Fasting Book and his pioneering philosophy on health. His daughter Patricia is a testament to the ageless value of living The Bragg Healthy Lifestyle. – Jay Robb, author of *The Fruit Flush*

During the many years Patricia worked with her father, she was right beside him, assisting him on Bragg Health Crusades worldwide. They were a great team, when you looked at them, you would see only two people headed in the same healthy direction!

I am a big fan of Paul Bragg. I fast and follow The Bragg Healthy Lifestyle daily. The world and I are blessed with the health teachings of Paul and Patricia Bragg!
– Tony Robbins • *TonyRobbins.com*

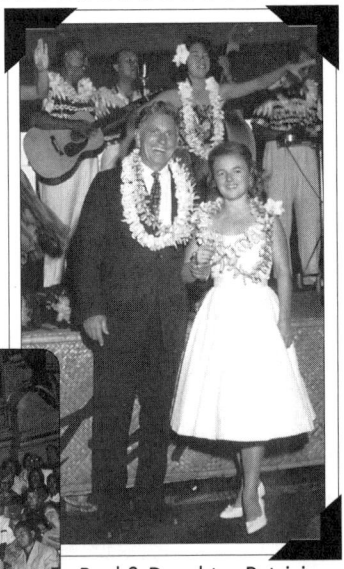

Paul & Daughter Patricia, Royal Hawaiian, Honolulu.

Dream big, think big and enjoy the many miracles.

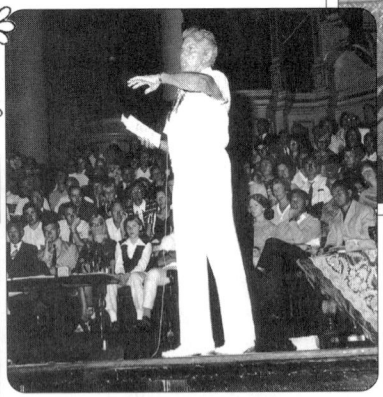

Paul – London Bragg Health Crusade.

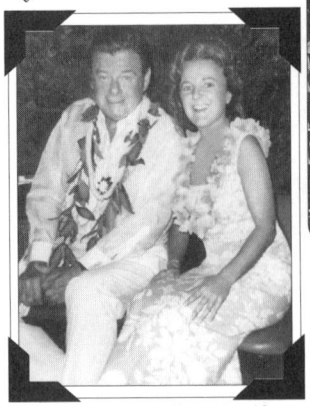

Actor Arthur Godfrey with Patricia, in Honolulu celebrating his 79th birthday.

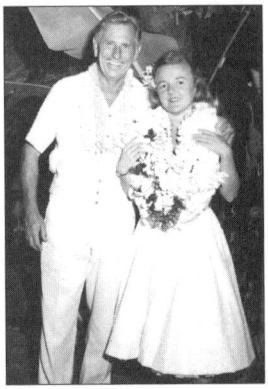

Health Crusaders Paul C. Bragg and daughter Patricia traveled the world spreading health, inspiring millions to renew and revitalize their health.

Bragg Mottos:
3 John 2 and Genesis 6:3

100 YEAR HISTORY OF BRAGG HEALTH BOOKS & PRODUCTS

PHOTO GALLERY

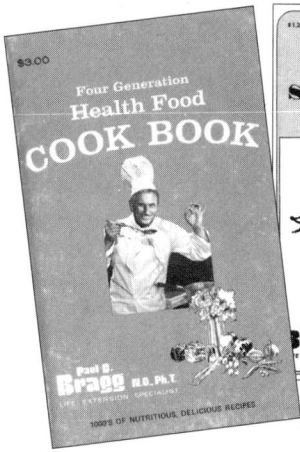

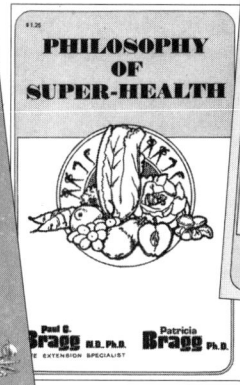

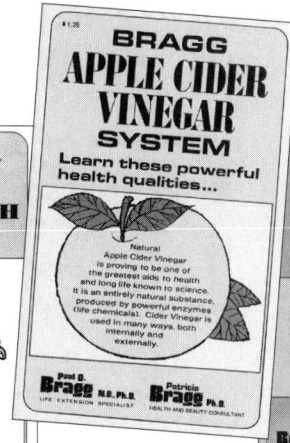

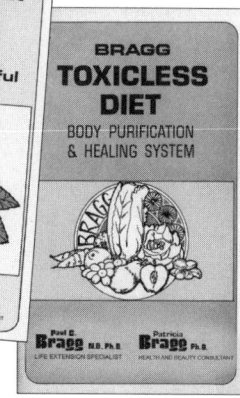

Paul and Patricia are passionate about spreading the message of health to the world.

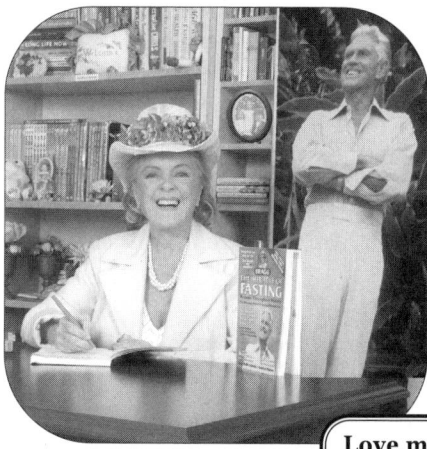

Patricia Bragg carries on her father's Health Legacy that he started over 100 years ago.

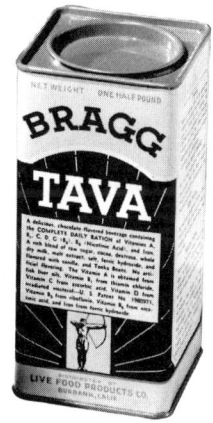

BRAGG TAVA
A delicious chocolate-flavored beverage. Contains vitamins A, B, C, B2, B6 and Iron.

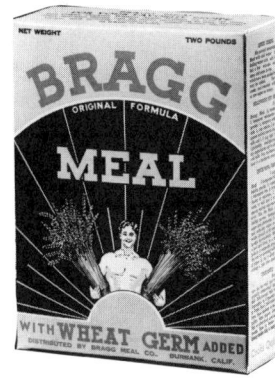

BRAGG MEAL CEREAL
Bragg was first to put wheat germ and 7 grains together for a delicious hot cereal.

Love makes the World go 'round.

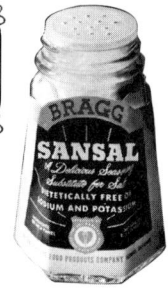

BRAGG SANSAL
A great Salt Substitute.
This product was approved by Los Angeles Heart Assoc.

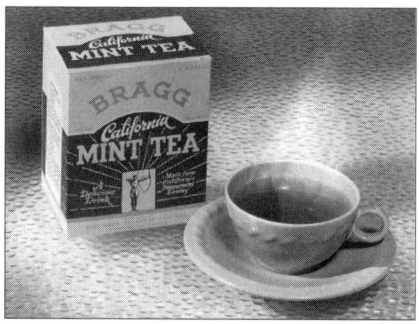

BRAGG ORGANIC MINT TEA
First Organic Herb Teas in America.

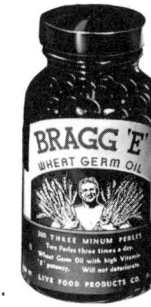

BRAGG 'E' WHEAT GERM OIL
Wheat germ oil with high Vitamin 'E' potency.
Includes Omega-3 and Omega-6.

"Our lives have completely turned around! Our family is feeling so healthy, we must tell you about it."– Gene & Joan Zollner, parents of 11, Washington

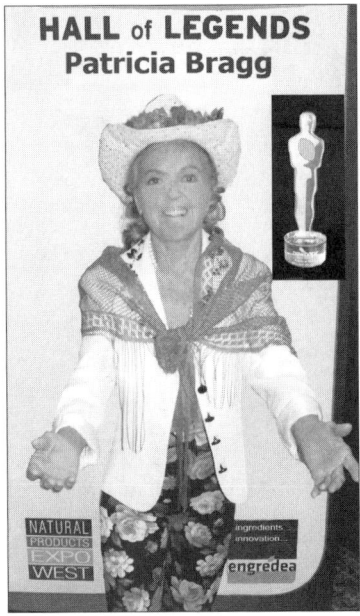

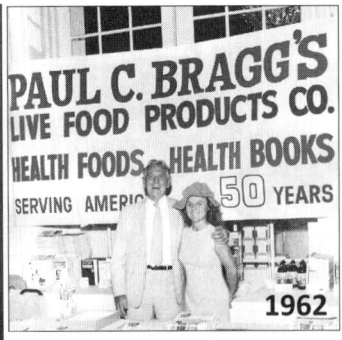

Paul C. Bragg with Patricia, celebrating over 50 years of Bragg Health Products, Books & Crusading worldwide, spreading Health around the world.

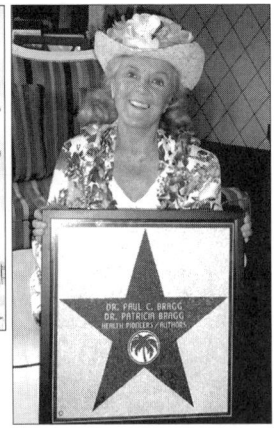

"Palm Spring Walk of Stars" – Patricia with Bragg Star.

Natural Foods Expo in Anaheim with 65,000 attendees from around the world honored Patricia Bragg and her father Paul C. Bragg as treasured Health Food Industry Legends.

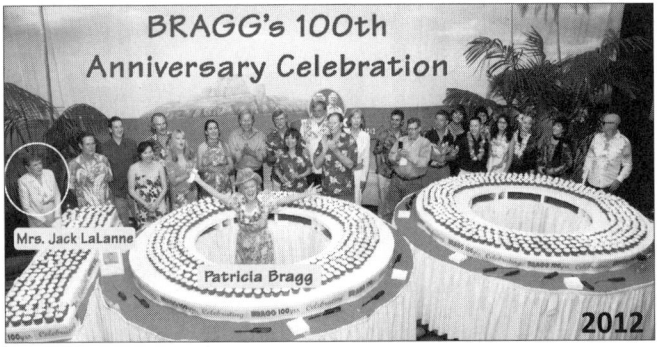

100 Year Anniversary Party celebrated at the Natural Foods Expo in Anaheim

Patricia, Staff & 1,000 Friends celebrated our 100 years of Bragg Healthy Products, Books & Health Crusading! We are proud Pioneers in this Big Health Industry that is helping to keep the world healthier! With Blessings of Health, Peace & Love to You!

Patricia

Bragg Hawaii Exercise Class was founded by Worldwide Health Crusader and Fitness Legend, Dr. Paul C. Bragg. He wanted to create a dynamic, Free Community Exercise Class, and he often taught these classes himself for many years. Patricia Bragg continues her father's health legacy by supporting the Bragg Exercise Class and participates in the class whenever she is in Hawaii.

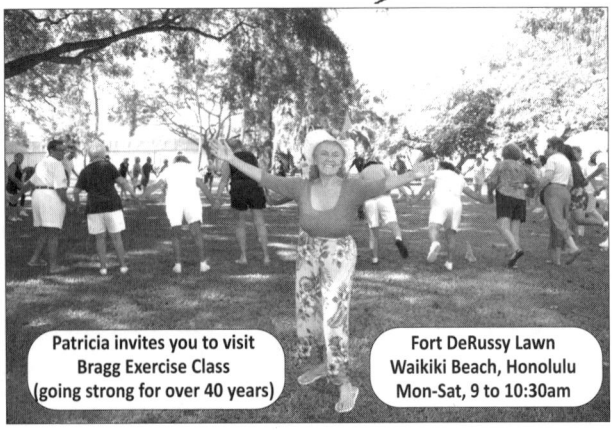

"Please make a record of your family history & background. Take pictures – make your own 'Photo Gallery'. Take videos – make movies of your children, spouse, mother and father, family gatherings, etc. These memories are precious & important to save for future generations." – Patricia Bragg

Index

A

Aches/Pains, 22, 23, 34, 45, 83, 89-91, 103, 118, 119, 163, 178, 180, 182, 184, 187, 189
Acupuncture/Acupressure, 165, 180, 186, 187, 190
Adrenaline, 36, 175
Ageing, 10, 11, 43, 57, 61, 110, 117, 118, 122, 137, 177
Aggression/Aggressive, 45, 53, 181
Alcohol, 15-17, 19, 24, 37, 39, 41, 42, 63, 68, 73, 74, 82, 94, 98, 153, 155, 157, 170, 177, 184
Alexander Technique, 189
Allergies, 91, 94, 103, 110, 137, 163
Alzheimer's Disease, 83, 84, 172, 184
Anger, 9, 26, 29, 36, 42, 127, 144, 145, 150, 151, 163, 173
Angina, 40, 84, 130, 171, 177
Antidepressants, 173, 181-183
Antioxidants, 91, 96, 98, 106, 122, 160, 184
Anxiety, 42, 53, 68, 83, 119, 136, 141, 153, 158, 160, 170, 173, 175, 176, 178-180
Aromatherapy, 72, 189
Arteries, 12, 29, 30, 32, 57, 91, 94, 115, 122, 137, 139, 157, 172
Arteriosclerosis, 30, 130
Arthritis, 89, 90, 92, 95, 102, 107, 118, 122, 181
Aspartame, 94, 163, 174
Asthma, 91, 107, 129, 131, 137, 158, 187
Attention Deficit Disorder, (ADD/ADHD) 161, 163, 170
Auto-immune Disease, 43, 158

B

Bacteria, 42, 91, 107, 137, 139, 185, 186
Beverages, 39, 41, 42, 70, 108, 180
Bipolar Disorder, 183
Bladder, 41, 137
Blood, 7, 20, 24, 29, 30, 32, 54, 65, 81, 83-86, 91, 93, 97, 98, 101, 102, 111, 113-115, 122, 123, 126, 130, 139, 147, 153, 158, 160, 169, 171, 173, 175-177, 180, 182-85, 187
Blood Pressure, 15, 29-31, 33, 89-91, 96, 110, 118, 121, 122, 130, 150, 153, 160, 171, 175-178
Blood Sugar, 39, 91, 113, 167, 176
Boron, 89, 160
Bowels, 7, 29, 40, 41, 83, 90, 95, 123, 165
Bragg Healthy Energy Smoothie, 106, 108 (recipe)
Bragg Healthy Lifestyle, xvi, 11, 12, 14, 16, 17, 19, 20, 22, 23, 30, 43, 48, 53, 56, 57, 59, 62, 77, 84, 94, 102, 104, 108, 110, 120, 133, 134, 160, 164, 191
Bragg, Patricia, A, B, D, E, H-N, iii, x, xvi, 5, 23, 25, 35, 36, 53, 75, 81, 80, 108, 110, 117, 120, 131, 133, 136, 164, 190-192, 220
Bragg, Paul, A-N, iii, vi, viii, ix, xvi, 6, 25, 58, 62, 110, 112, 116, 117, 120, 121, 134, 136, 140, 148, 188-190, 192
Brain, 1-3, 19, 20, 32, 33, 38, 42, 56, 65-68, 71, 72, 77, 81, 83, 90, 95-98, 101, 111, 114, 131, 140, 160, 162, 166, 167, 169-172, 175, 177, 181-185

Index

B continued

Breathing, 6, 11, 14, 20, 21, 24, 25, 32, 33, 38, 50, 72, 74, 124,-133, 136, 138, 158, 159, 179, 188

C

Cabbage, 40, 68, 85, 87, 91, 99, 106-109
Caffeine, 17, 19, 24, 37, 39, 42, 63, 67, 68, 73, 74, 76, 81, 82, 94, 103, 153, 155, 157, 162, 164, 179
Calcium, 31, 53, 67, 73, 78, 80, 85-90, 95, 97, 122, 153, 160, 162, 165, 170-172, 175, 176, 178
Cancer, 30, 39, 42-43, 80, 89, 91, 92, 105, 107, 115, 119, 122, 130, 137-139, 141, 160, 161, 172, 176, 177
Candida, 32, 164, 185
Capillaries, 76, 91
Carbohydrates, 97, 113, 175, 181, 185
Cardiovascular Disease, 33, 40, 84, 172, 176
Cataracts, 122, 130
Cayenne (capsaicin), 85, 108, 122, 171
Chelation Therapy, 172
Children/Youth, 5, 12, 13, 15, 17, 31, 44, 63, 77, 86, 88, 105, 112, 122, 125, 127, 130, 144, 147, 157, 161-163, 166-167, 180
Chiropractic, 122, 157, 165, 187
Chlorine, 137-139
Cholesterol, 15, 29-31, 54, 80, 88, 91, 94, 98, 110, 119, 122, 137-139, 153, 160, 172
Chondroitin, 122
Chromosomes, 43
Chronic Fatigue (CFS), 11, 161, 163-165, 185
CIP Method, 33
Circulation, 11, 24, 25, 33, 57, 64, 65, 102, 111, 114, 115, 126, 134, 146, 184, 187, 190
Cleansing, 7, 13, 15, 24, 102, 110, 129, 133, 187
Coffee, *(see caffeine)*
Constipation, 11, 15, 40, 71, 127, 156

D

Dairy, 78, 80, 88, 92, 99, 100, 103, 105, 180
Dementia, 43, 111
Depression, 3, 29, 39-40, 43, 70, 71, 83, 85, 89, 90, 95, 112, 113, 119, 147, 160, 164, 168, 170, 172, 176-178, 181-183, 185
Detoxification, 91, 102, 186
Diabetes, 15, 30, 31, 39-40, 43, 80, 83, 90, 95, 96, 105, 115, 119, 130, 141, 165, 167, 172
Diet, 15, 17, 19, 24, 30, 31, 37, 39, 40, 42, 44, 63, 67, 77-82, 84, 85, 87, 90, 95, 101-110, 122, 150, 161, 162, 164-170, 173, 177, 180, 181, 185, 188
Digestion, 7, 38-42, 68, 96, 102, 122, 127, 145
Dopamine, 181, 184
Drugs/Medications, 19, 33, 37, 39, 42, 74, 76, 77, 82, 83, 94, 98, 130, 146, 153, 157, 160, 177, 178, 182, 188

There is no failure except the failure of trying. – Elbert Hubbard

Index

E

Elimination, 102, 103, 110, 122, 127, 133
Emotional Health, 42, 116, 191
Emotions, 2, 24, 25, 32, 36, 39-40, 45, 49, 51-53, 86, 89, 111, 112, 114, 116, 127, 136, 143-147, 150, 151, 175, 182, 184
Emphysema, 130, 158, 187
Energy, 5, 19, 30, 34, 36, 37, 40, 42, 45, 47-51, 56, 60, 62, 64, 69, 75, 82, 83, 96, 97, 102, 103, 114, 119, 140, 142, 144, 150, 154, 158, 164, 167, 175, 179, 183, 184, 187-189, 191
Epstein-Barr, 163
Essential Fatty Acids, 78, 90, 92, 183-185
Exercise, 6, 11, 14, 20, 22, 24, 25, 30, 31, 40, 44, 53, 56, 63, 65-68, 73, 76, 84, 89, 111-122, 125, 134, 136, 140, 142, 144, 147, 149, 156, 157, 159, 160, 162, 164-166, 173, 177, 179, 187, 188, 190, 192
Eyes, 57, 74, 90, 91, 103, 129, 139, 142, 160

F

Faith, 25, 47, 52-54, 57, 61-62, 110, 136
Fasting, 11, 14, 16, 17, 24, 25, 36, 102, 110, 118, 133, 189
Fat, 29-31, 80, 88, 89, 94, 98, 105, 120, 122, 157, 175, 184
Fatigue, 7, 37, 82, 90, 153, 162, 164, 169
Fears, 9, 21, 24, 25, 29, 38, 45, 47, 53, 55-62, 123, 136, 140, 146, 151, 158, 179
Feet, 33, 72, 86, 90, 188
Feldenkrais Method, 189
Fiber, 40, 68, 89, 92, 105, 122, 165
Flaxseed, 91, 98, 106
Fluoridation, 138
Folic Acid (Folate), 83, 84, 122, 160, 165
Foods, 24, 25, 30, 31, 37, 39-44, 56, 63, 67, 68, 73, 77-93, 96, 101-110, 118, 119, 122, 133, 136, 139, 142, 162, 164, 166-168, 171, 178, 180, 181, 184
Foods to Avoid (list), 94
Framingham Heart Study, 29, 117, 118, 144
Free Radicals, 122, 176
Fruits, 24, 30, 40, 72, 78, 79, 84, 85, 89-94, 98, 99, 103, 105, 108, 113, 119, 122, 162, 164, 177, 181
Fungus, 185, 186

G

Garlic, 91, 93, 108, 109, 122, 165, 171, 185
Ginger, 180
Ginkgo Biloba, 98, 165, 176, 179, 184, 185
Glucosamine, 122
Grains, 30, 78-79, 79, 85, 89, 90, 93, 95, 97-99, 103, 105, 122, 164, 171
Grape Seed Extract, 122
Gratitude, 151
Grief, 9, 15, 26, 53, 127, 149, 150, 172
Gums/Gum Disease, 177, 186

Index

H

Habits, 11, 16, 25, 36, 47, 68, 77, 78, 82, 86, 110, 118, 119, 122, 136, 154, 155, 157, 166, 184, 191
Happiness, 6, 12-14, 16, 21, 25, 34, 35, 48, 50, 53, 61, 72, 75, 77, 87, 104, 110, 126, 128, 136, 141, 146-151, 158-161, 179, 181
HDL (good cholesterol), 30, 122
Headaches, 15, 45, 83, 90, 103, 163-164, 178, 180, 182
Healthy Heart Habits (list), 122
Heart Attack, 30, 32, 40, 93, 144
Heart Disease, 15, 29, 30, 71, 80, 84, 89, 91, 92, 105, 118, 119, 137, 150, 165, 172, 177
Heart Palpitations, 45, 86, 179
Heimlich Maneuver, 131
Herbs, 85, 93, 98, 109, 157, 171, 179, 188, 190
Hiking, 111, 112, 115-116, 149, 159, 160
Hippocrates, xii, 143, 170, 192
Homeopathy, 188
Homocysteine, 83, 84, 110, 122, 153, 160
Hormones, 42, 89, 91, 94, 166, 175, 176
Hospitals, 44, 62
Hyperactive, 161, 162, 167
Hypertension, 29-32, 130, 178
Hypoglycemia, 167

I

Immune System, 15, 34, 71, 83, 91, 107, 119, 122, 123, 137, 142, 158, 163-165, 176, 177
Inflammation, 15, 42-43, 79, 90, 95, 118
Insomnia, 15, 67-74, 83, 110, 160, 168, 178, 179, 182
Insulin, 39-40, 42, 165, 167
Irritable Bowel Syndrome, 90
Isoflavones, 91 (chart)

J

Joints, 83, 89, 102, 118, 119, 122, 163, 164, 172, 181, 182
Juices, 79, 92, 94, 100, 108, 110, 122, 162, 164
Junk Foods, 19, 31, 41, 78, 161, 164, 167, 171

K

Kidneys, 7, 114, 123, 171
Koop, Dr. C. Everett, 81

L

LaLanne, Jack/Elaine, B, F, H, K, 109, 120
LDL (bad cholesterol), 29, 30, 122
Lecithin, 98, 122, 165
Lemon Balm, 53, 70, 73, 180
Lentils, 80, 85, 92, 96-99, 106, 107, 109

Your Daily Habits Form Your Future

Habits can be wrong, good or bad, healthy or unhealthy, rewarding or unrewarding. The right or wrong habits, decisions, actions, words or deeds . . . are up to you! Wisely choose your habits, as they can make or break your life! – Patricia Bragg

Index

Lifestyle, 6, 8, 11, 21, 31, 33, 36, 39, 44, 45, 48, 51, 59, 65, 73, 75, 78, 79, 89, 98, 100, 118, 140, 154, 157, 164, 179, 191, 192
Liver, 7, 72, 91, 101, 114, 127, 137, 168, 181, 182
Longevity, 13, 22, 78, 80, 93, 111, 122, 141, 192
Lungs, 7, 24, 40, 101, 111, 114, 119, 123-126, 129-131, 139, 146, 149, 158
Lymph Nodes, 163, 186

M

Magnesium, 31, 53, 67, 70, 73, 89, 95, 97, 122, 153, 160, 162, 165, 169-171, 176
Massage, 70, 72, 134, 157, 158, 165, 186-190
Mattress, 64, 73, 74, 76
Meat, 41, 80, 84, 89, 94, 96, 103, 178, 180
Meditation, 11, 12, 14, 17, 19, 21, 24, 39, 44, 47-57, 72, 128, 159, 190
Mediterranean Diet, 93, 173
Melatonin, 53, 70-73, 122, 165, 176
Memory, 2, 57, 71, 73, 90, 91, 98, 122, 149, 163, 167, 183, 184
Mental Energy/Sharpness, 119
Mental Illness, 8, 44, 110, 168
Metabolism, 37, 48, 88, 91, 98, 100, 102, 137, 158, 165, 184
Migraines, 15, 174, 180, 187
Milk, 88, 89, 92, 103, 105, 168
Minerals, 31, 81, 85-87, 89, 90, 92, 97, 160, 162, 167, 169, 178
Moods/Moodiness, 42, 45, 67, 71, 85, 86, 103, 113, 120, 147, 158, 181-184

N

Naturopathy, 188
Negative Thoughts, 20, 21, 24, 34, 49, 50, 173
Nerve Depletion, 3, 40-42, 44
Nerve Depression, 3
Nerve Exhaustion, 9, 37, 41, 44, 56, 81, 123, 143
Nerve Force, 1, 2, 5-20, 24, 29, 34, 36, 37, 39, 40, 45, 47, 48, 50-52, 54-60, 62, 63, 76, 77, 81, 82, 85, 87, 111, 114, 123, 128, 133-136, 140-146, 148-153, 155-157, 159, 191
Nerve Tension, 3, 29, 62, 123, 127
Nerves, 3, 5-7, 9, 14, 15, 18, 22, 25, 33, 37, 40-42, 44-45, 51, 53, 66, 70, 85, 86, 102, 114, 122, 126-128, 134, 136, 140-142, 145, 146, 153, 154, 156, 157, 160, 169-170, 180, 191
Nervous System, 1, 2, 3, 7, 18, 21, 25, 29, 32, 33, 38-42, 44, 47, 63, 64, 68, 77, 78, 81, 90, 114, 123, 127, 129, 136, 140, 142, 143, 149, 157, 154, 156, 170, 172, 176, 179, 183, 187, 188
Nervousness, 11, 15, 16, 45, 82, 86, 87, 135, 140, 170
Nutrition, 6, 9, 20, 25, 31, 77, 78, 80, 81, 88, 94, 97, 100, 136, 140, 162, 165-168, 188, 192

O

Obesity, 15, 31, 43, 119, 172, 177
Oil Pulling, 186
Oils, 92, 94, 103, 186
Omega-3, 80, 90, 95, 122, 173, 181, 183

Index

O continued

Organic Foods, 24, 30, 40, 78-80, 84, 89, 92, 94-96, 105-109, 119, 122, 142, 162, 164, 170, 171
Ornish, Dean, M.D. 12,
Osteoarthritis, 122, 182
Osteopathy, 188
Osteoporosis, 83, 84, 89, 118, 119, 130, 160, 171
Oxygen, 9, 24, 32, 63, 98, 111, 112, 114, 115, 123, 128, 130, 158

P

Panic/Panic Attacks, 21, 38, 42, 45, 179
Pesticides, 103
Phosphorus, 88, 89, 176
Phytochemicals, 80, 90, 91(chart)
Posture, 11, 22, 23, 25, 85, 119, 136, 160, 187-189
Potassium, 31, 81, 90, 165, 170, 171, 175, 177, 178
Premature ageing, 43, 57, 61
Prevention, 31, 32, 78, 190
Protein, 68, 72, 78, 80, 92, 95, 97, 99 (chart), 137, 162, 164, 175, 181
Pulse, 48, 67, 103, 127, 128

R

Recipes, 67, 108, 109, 180
Refined Foods, 40, 96, 164, 170, 184
Reflexology Therapy, 188
Reiki Therapy, 189
Relaxation, 11, 13, 14, 21, 25, 26, 32-34, 49, 63, 64, 74-76, 141, 153-158, 180, 189, 190
Rolfing Therapy, 189

S

Salads, 79, 89, 92-94, 96, 103, 106, 107, 109, 122, 185
Salt/Sodium, 43, 89, 93, 94, 103, 105, 157, 165, 170, 177-178, 184
SAMe, 165, 176, 179-182, 184
Seizures, 174, 183
Serotonin, 21, 42, 67, 71, 72, 181
Shiatsu Therapy, 190
Shower, 70, 72, 76, 133, 134, 137-139, 188
Skin, 1, 7, 15, 32, 37, 76, 85, 133-135, 137-139, 141, 142, 160, 176, 188, 189
Skin Brushing, 134, 188
Sleep, 9, 11, 24-26, 48, 53, 61, 63-76, 103, 114, 119, 122, 136, 140, 163, 165-166, 175, 179

When you sell a man a book you don't just sell him paper, ink and glue, you sell him a whole new life! There's heaven and earth in a real book, and the main purpose of books is to trap the mind into its own thinking and action.
– Christopher Morley, Honored American Journalist and Poet

Touch is a primal need, as necessary for growth as food, clothing or shelter. Michelangelo knew this when he painted God extending a hand toward Adam on ceiling of Sistine Chapel, he chose touch to depict the gift of life.
– George H. Colt, American Journalist, Author "The Big House"

Index

Smoking, 110, 126, 127, 129, 130, 142, 179
Soy, 72, 80, 91, 92, 98, 99, 105, 122, 164, 171, 181
Sports Massage, 190
St. John's Wort, 165, 176, 179, 182, 184
Stevia, 68, 94, 107, 108, 180
Stress, 2, 5, 9, 15, 24, 26 (test), 29, 32-38, 40, 54, 62, 63, 69, 71, 72, 74, 77, 81, 90, 111, 112, 114, 119, 127, 134, 136, 141, 143, 144, 148, 150, 154-156, 158, 160, 168, 170, 175-187, 189, 190
Stretching, 22, 158, 165, 179, 189
Stroke, 15, 29, 30, 32, 91, 105, 119, 177, 185, 190
Sugar, 42, 63, 67, 72, 73, 82, 89, 94, 96, 105, 122, 162, 164, 165, 167, 173, 174, 178, 180, 185
Suicide, 15, 16, 19, 42, 61, 82, 151
Sunshine, 12, 21, 76, 89, 111, 141, 142, 147, 150, 151, 160, 166
Surgery, 188
Swedish Massage Therapy, 190

T

Teeth, 57, 85, 101, 186
Telomeres, 43-44
Therapies, Alternative, 54, 72, 89, 157, 162, 165, 169, 172, 183, 186, 187, 188, 189, 190, 192
Throat, 73, 129, 132, 139, 163, 186
Thyroid, 114, 124, 172, 175
TMS (Transcranial Magnetic Stimulation), 173, 183
Tobacco/Nicotine, 19, 24, 42, 63, 73, 76, 82, 129, 130, 153, 157
Tragering Therapy, 189
Tuberculosis, 6

V

Vegetables, 24, 30, 40, 78, 79, 84, 85, 89, 90, 92-96, 98, 99, 103, 105, 108-109, 119, 122, 162, 164-165, 171, 177, 181
Vegetarian, 17, 92, 93, 99, 105, 141, 162
Violence/Crime, 65, 66, 130, 144
Vision, 52, 174
Vitamins, 53, 77-82, 84, 85, 88, 89, 92, 97, 122, 126, 141, 160, 162, 165, 167-170, 173, 176, 183
Vitamin A, 88, 160, 165
Vitamin B, 21, 53, 77, 78, 80, 82-85, 90, 92, 95, 97, 160, 162, 165, 169, 170, 176, 183, 184
Vitamin C, 84, 106, 108, 122, 160, 162, 165
Vitamin D, 78, 88, 89, 126, 141, 142, 160, 165
Vitamin E, 90, 92, 95, 122, 162, 165

A gift is pure when it is given from the heart to the right person at the right time and at the right place and when we expect nothing in return.

I am beginning to learn that it is the sweet, simple things of life which are the real ones after all. – Laura Ingalls Wilder, Author, 1867-1957

Index

W

Waistline, 120
Walking, 20, 22, 24, 67, 111-115, 122, 149, 173
Water, 16, 24, 25, 41, 67, 78-79, 84, 97, 100-102, 108, 110, 113, 131, 133-140, 158, 164, 168, 188, 189
Water Therapy, 134-136, 140, 188
Weight Lifting, 89, 117, 118
Weight Loss, 37, 90, 96, 110, 119, 177
Wheat, 79, 85-90, 94, 95, 99, 103, 107, 170, 171
Wheat Germ, 85, 98, 99, 106, 170

Y

Yoga, 21, 38, 44, 67, 113, 158, 190
Youthful, 22, 56, 58, 62, 114, 117, 120, 161

Z

Zinc, 97, 102, 122, 165, 168, 171, 176
Zone/Reflexology Therapy, 188

Dream big, think big & enjoy the many miracles.

WE THANK THEE

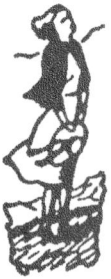

For flowers that bloom about our feet;
For song of bird and hum of bee;
For all things fair we hear or see,
Father in heaven we thank Thee!

For blue of stream and blue of sky;
For pleasant shade of branches high;
For fragrant air and cooling breeze;
For beauty of the blooming trees,
Father in heaven we thank Thee!

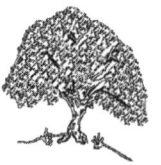

For mother love and father care;
For brothers strong and sisters fair;
For love at home and here each day;
For guidance lest we go astray,
Father in heaven we thank Thee!

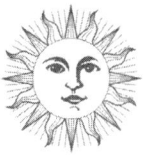

For this new morning with its light;
For rest and shelter of the night;
For health and food, for love and friends;
For every thing His goodness sends
Father in heaven we thank Thee!

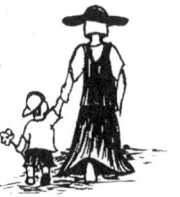

~ Ralph Waldo Emerson

BRAGG "HOW-TO, SELF-HEALTH" BOOKS

Authored by America's First Family of Health

Live Longer – Healthier – Stronger Self-Improvement Library

Apple Cider Vinegar - Miracle Health System

BY PAUL C. BRAGG, N.D., PH.D.
and PATRICIA BRAGG

Paul C. Bragg, originator of health stores in America, and world-renowned health crusader Patricia Bragg, introduced America to the life-changing value of Apple Cider Vinegar, with the miracle enzyme known as "the mother." Now a widely popular beverage, this book reveals the legendary health-and life-giving versatility of apple cider vinegar. Following in the footsteps of Hippocrates, who taught the benefits of ACV to his patients in 400 BC, the Braggs teach dozens of reasons to use vinegar, including as a beauty aid, for skin treatments, in recipes, as an antibiotic, anti-septic, hair-revitalizing rinse, headache reliever, and weight reducer. ACV optimizes digestive health and can reduce or eliminate acid reflux. Paul and Patricia Bragg have helped millions heal and restore their vitality and zest for life through their time-tested understanding of natural health. *Apple Cider Vinegar: Miracle Health System* is informative, entertaining, and invaluable for anyone wanting to feel their best.

Bragg Healthy Lifestyle - Vital Living at Any Age

BY PAUL C. BRAGG, N.D., PH.D.
and PATRICIA BRAGG

Learn the simple strategies of radical health and vibrant wellness that The Bragg Healthy Lifestyle has brought to millions! What is an ageless body? For health pioneers Paul C. Bragg and Patricia Bragg, an ageless body sparkles with vitality, immune strength, mental clarity, and digestive ease. The Braggs teach why a toxic-free diet maximizes energy, supports weight loss, and can help heal illness and disease. In the newly revised *Bragg Healthy Lifestyle: Vital Living At Any Age*, the trailblazing father-daughter team who alerted us nearly a century ago to the dangers of sugar and toxic foods, detail every key aspect of creating and maintaining ageless health, including detoxification, stress-release, nutrition, exercise and the importance of taking charge of not only what goes into our bodies, but practices such as fasting, which release the toxins that may unnecessarily accelerate the aging process. "You are what you eat, drink, breathe, think, say and do," is the Bragg motto. From the foods we eat to our outlook, the environments we live in and even in our physical activities, the authors encourage readers to replace toxins with nutrients, flush out poisons and waste efficiently, exercise, breathe deeply and well, and cultivate happiness and harmony in our daily lives.

Bragg Books are available at most Health & Book Stores – Nationwide

HEALTH SCIENCE
7127 Hollister Avenue, Suite 25A, Box 249, Santa Barbara, CA 93117
Toll-Free: (833) 408-1122

BRAGG "HOW-TO, SELF-HEALTH" BOOKS

Authored by America's First Family of Health

Live Longer – Healthier – Stronger Self-Improvement Library

The Miracle of Fasting - Proven Throughout History

BY PAUL C. BRAGG, N.D., PH.D.
and PATRICIA BRAGG

In this newly revised best-seller, known to millions as the "bible of fasting" health pioneers and researchers Paul C. Bragg and Patricia Bragg teach why this ancient practice is key to health and energy, and critical to longevity and ageless vitality, due to our toxic environment and the stress of our daily lives. They share a detailed, step-by-step approach, accessible and informative for both beginners and experienced fasters. Our bodies must process not only our food and water, but the air we breathe, and whatever chemicals they may contain. Since detoxification and digestion take more energy than even strenuous athletic pursuits, fasting allows the mind and body to rest, renew and regenerate, to come into harmony and balance, and release the effects of stimulating foods like caffeine and sugars. The goal of fasting, say the authors, is to allow for the mind and body to self-heal. This concise, tightly edited *The Miracle of Fasting* is filled with personal stories of Paul C. Bragg's travels around the world, including a fasting journey in India with Mahatma Gandhi.

Healthy Heart - Learn the Facts

BY PAUL C. BRAGG, N.D., PH.D.
and PATRICIA BRAGG

Heart disease claims more American lives than any other illness and is the number one cause of death for women. World-renowned health pioneers Paul C. Bragg and Patricia Bragg teach time-tested, proven strategies for healing and maintaining a healthy heart for a long, active life! In a world filled with technological wizardry and products, the human heart still outperforms them all. That is – if that human heart is kept healthy. That is what the trailblazers Paul C. Bragg and Patricia Bragg have done in this book, sharing simple suggestions for lifestyle changes, nutritional support and exercises that will keep this most miraculous machine, your body, healthy and strong. You will learn how the heart works and how and why coronary disease is preventable and reversible. The authors provide an easy-to-follow blueprint for heart health that includes stress-release techniques, affirming that a positive mental outlook on life is a major element of heart health. The Braggs are legendary in the field of nutrition and health, and this newly revised and edited edition is a foundation of The Bragg Healthy Lifestyle. It is one of the most comprehensive heart health books on the market today.

Bragg Books are available at most Health & Book Stores – Nationwide

HEALTH SCIENCE
7127 Hollister Avenue, Suite 25A, Box 249, Santa Barbara, CA 93117
Toll-Free: (833) 408-1122

Authored by America's First Family of Health

Live Longer – Healthier – Stronger Self-Improvement Library

Building Powerful Nerve Force & Positive Energy - Reduce Stress, Worry and Anger

BY PAUL C. BRAGG, N.D., PH.D.
and PATRICIA BRAGG

What is Nerve Force and why should you care about it? According to mental health trailblazers Paul C. Bragg and Patricia Bragg, "Nerve Force" is a type of life energy stored in the nerves, muscles, organs, and brain. The more Nerve Force you have, the quicker you can re-charge it, and the healthier, happier, and more satisfying a life you will lead. If you suffer from burnout, stress, fatigue, anxiety, insomnia or depression, this book is for you! We know that the ability to feel joy and peace is essential to a complete experience of vitality and wellness. Our thoughts, our attitudes, our outlook, and our emotional well-being are all dependent on having a powerful "Nerve Force." Just like any muscle that we can develop and strengthen, we can build our Nerve Force so that we are resilient, relaxed, and calm, even during times of stress. Paul C. Bragg and Patricia Bragg show you how with simple mental exercises and suggestions for specific foods that replenish your Nerve Force, as well as foods that deplete it, in this newly revised edition of *Building Powerful Nerve Force & Positive Energy* the father-daughter team explains to readers the reward of paying attention to the energy that is responsible for not only our physical capabilities and our vital body functions, but our ability to process information and feel centered and grounded, no matter what life throws at us. They teach us that maintaining a healthy Nerve Force, leads to a balanced and fruitful life.

Super Power Breathing - For Optimum Health & Healing

BY PAUL C. BRAGG, N.D., PH.D.
and PATRICIA BRAGG

Do you sometimes find that you are panting instead of breathing? Many of us do! This can cause headaches, anxiety, fatigue, and brain fog. The quality of our breath determines the quality of our life! This book teaches us how to breathe in a way that replenishes the body with the oxygen it so deeply craves. "The more effectively we breathe, the more effectively we live," write the authors, world-renowned health pioneers Paul C. Bragg and Patricia Bragg. "Super Power Breathing can make your life-force stronger, calmer and smarter." The Super Power Breathing program has been followed by Olympic athletes and millions of Bragg followers, and is filled with simple exercises for energizing and rejuvenating your breath, and your whole body. Research shows that we use only one-fourth to one-half of our lung capacity with each breath. This starves our body much like if we are depriving it of food. We are slowly robbing our body of its most vital, invisible nourishment – oxygen. In its newly revised form, the Bragg Super Power Breathing Program will give you all the tools you need to shift from shallow breathing to taking deep, oxygen-filled, life-giving breaths!

Authored by America's First Family of Health

Live Longer – Healthier – Stronger Self-Improvement Library

Water - The Shocking Truth

BY PAUL C. BRAGG, N.D., PH.D.
and PATRICIA BRAGG

The water you drink can literally make or break your health. The purity of our water is the most critical element in maintaining radical vitality, and healing from illness and disease. In this newly revised edition of *Water: The Shocking Truth*, health crusaders Paul C. Bragg and Patricia Bragg reveal the dangers of tap water, which research shows can be responsible for many ailments, due to the addition of dangerous chemicals such as fluoride and chlorine. In this book, the trailblazing father-daughter team teach the many functions water performs in the body, from regulating the various systems to flushing the body of waste and toxins. But what if the substance we use to cleanse our bodies is itself polluted? With the mandatory fluoridation of water in the municipal water systems, the authors assert that has been the case for decades. Added to the public water supply to prevent tooth decay starting in the 1950s, fluoride has long been known to be a toxin, used in pesticides and rat poisons. Learn what types of water are optimal to drink, how and why to detox your body with nature's most life-giving liquid, and the health-and-life-saving value of installing a water filter in your shower!

Bragg Back & Foot Fitness Program - Keys to a Pain-Free Back & Strong Healthy Feet

BY PAUL C. BRAGG, N.D., PH.D.
and PATRICIA BRAGG

If you are suffering with back or foot pain, look no further for a comprehensive program that will restore health to the parts of your body that carry you through life! Remember when we were children, and we had the kind of energy and flexibility to play for hours? Agile and active, we could twist, bend, stretch and climb with little effort. However, hours looking at a computer screen, a sedentary lifestyle and poor posture can take their toll. Eventually our backs start to hurt and cramp with every movement, and our feet ache after just a short walk. We start feeling "old." In *Bragg Back & Foot Fitness Program*, the father-daughter team of world-renowned health pioneers, Paul C. Bragg and Patricia Bragg teach how to speed the healing of injuries and develop a strong and flexible back and healthy feet, rejuvenating and re-energizing our bodies in the process. The trailblazing health experts who brought wellness and vitality to millions, including fitness guru Jack LaLanne, outline the keys to a healthy spine, pain-free back and bunion-free feet through nutritional support and clearly illustrated, simple exercises, as well as other tips for posture and massage. Paul and Patricia Bragg reveal the healing properties of herbs, effective ways to practice foot reflexology, how to deal with arthritis, athlete's foot, plantar fasciitis, and foot problems caused by diabetes. By following the authors' Back and Foot Care Program, you can begin to treat your body as Mother Nature intended you to, and creating painless feet, a strong back and a powerful body will begin!

PATRICIA BRAGG

Health Crusader and "Angel of Health and Healing"

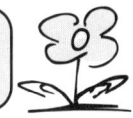

Author, Lecturer, Nutritionist, Health & Lifestyle Educator to World Leaders, Hollywood Stars, Singers, Athletes & Millions.

Patricia is a life-long health advocate and activist, admired internationally for her passionate work promoting healthy living. For many years she traveled the world, teaching The Bragg Healthy Lifestyle for physical, spiritual, emotional health and joy. She was invited to give lectures, visited radio shows, was profiled in magazines and appealed to people of all ages, nationalities and walks-of-life. Together with Paul, she co-authored a collection of ten books, with inspiration and techniques for living a long, vital, happy life. Now in her 90s and living on an organic farm in California, Patricia herself is a testament to these teachings and the sparkling symbol of health, perpetual youth and radiant energy.

PAUL C. BRAGG, N.D., Ph.D.

Life Extension Specialist • World Health Crusader
Lecturer and Advisor to Olympic Athletes, Royalty, Stars & Millions.
Originator of Health Food Stores & Founder of Health Movement Worldwide

Paul C. Bragg was at the forefront of the modern health movement, having inspired generations to turn toward wellness. At a young age, Paul turned his own health around by developing an eating, breathing and exercise program to build strength and vitality. From this life-changing experience, he pledged to dedicate the rest of his life to promoting a healthy lifestyle. He opened one of the country's first health food stores, which eventually led to the creation of the Bragg Live Foods company. With a devoted following, Paul traveled giving lectures and sharing his expertise, while serving as an advisor to athletes and movie stars alike. Even Jack LaLanne, the original television fitness guru, credited Paul with having introduced him to the importance of healthy living. In addition to the books Paul wrote with Patricia, they co-hosted television and radio shows and worked together to bring wellness to the world. Paul himself excelled in athletics, loved the ocean and the outdoors, and radiated with health and a warm smile.

Patricia inspires you to Renew, Rejuvenate and Revitalize your Life with "The Bragg Healthy Lifestyle" Books. Millions have benefitted from these life-changing philosophies with a longer, healthier, happier life!

Take Time for 12 Things

1. Take time to **Work** –
   it is the price of success.
2. Take time to **Think** –
   it is the source of power.
3. Take time to **Play** –
   it is the secret of youth.
4. Take time to **Read** –
   it is the foundation of knowledge.
5. Take time to **Worship** –
   it is the highway of reverence and washes the dust of earth from our eyes.
6. Take time to **Help and Enjoy Friends** –
   it is the source of happiness.
7. Take time to **Love and Share** –
   it is the one sacrament of life.
8. Take time to **Dream** –
   it hitches the soul to the stars.
9. Take time to **Laugh** –
   it is the singing that helps life's loads.
10. Take time for **Beauty** –
    it is everywhere in nature.
11. Take time for **Health** –
    it is the true wealth and treasure of life.
12. Take time to **Plan** –
    it is the secret of being able to have time for the first 11 things.

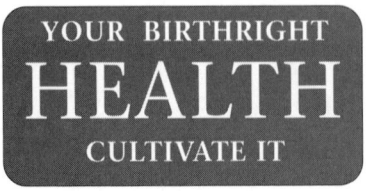

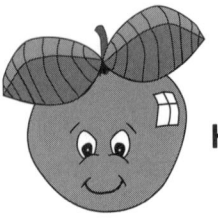

Have an Apple Healthy Life!

3 John 2

Teach me thy way, LORD, lead me in a straight path, because of my oppressors. – Psalm 27:11